Working with Deaf People – a Handbook for
Healthcare Professionals

D1336318

Working with Deaf People – a Handbook for Healthcare Professionals

Edited by **Anna Middleton**

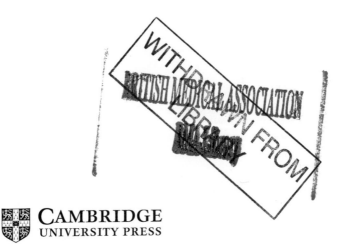

CAMBRIDGE
UNIVERSITY PRESS

CAMBRIDGE UNIVERSITY PRESS
Cambridge, New York, Melbourne, Madrid, Cape Town, Singapore,
São Paulo, Delhi, Dubai, Tokyo

Cambridge University Press
The Edinburgh Building, Cambridge CB2 8RU, UK

Published in the United States of America by
Cambridge University Press, New York

www.cambridge.org
Information on this title: www.cambridge.org/9780521690850

First published 2010

Printed in the United Kingdom at the University Press, Cambridge

A catalogue record for this publication is available from the British Library

Library of Congress Cataloguing in Publication data
Working with deaf people : a handbook for healthcare professionals /
  Anna Middleton (editor).
     p. ; cm.
  Includes bibliographical references and index.
  ISBN 978-0-521-69085-0 (pbk.)
  1. Medical personnel and patient–Handbooks, manuals, etc.
  2. Deaf–Medical care–Handbooks, manuals, etc. I. Middleton, Anna. II. Title.
  [DNLM: 1. Communication. 2. Professional-Patient Relations.
  3. Hearing Impaired Persons. W 62 W926 2010]
  R727.3.W67 2010
  362.4′2–dc22
  2009035489

ISBN 978-0-521-69085-0 Paperback

Additional resources for this publication at
www.cambridge.org/9780521690850

CONTENTS

GLOSSARY

ABI	Auditory brainstem implant, one of the treatment options for clients with NF2
A + E	Accident and Emergency department in a hospital
ASL	American Sign Language
BDA	British Deaf Association
BSL	British Sign Language
CHARGE	A genetic condition which causes deafblindness as well as heart and development problems
CRS	Congenital rubella syndrome, a cause of deafblindness
DDA	Disability Discrimination Act, legislation in the UK
*d*eaf	Could be used generically to describe all people with any level or perception of deafness or could be used by those who are profoundly deaf. Could be used by deaf people who use speech and/or sign language

Deaf	Used by deaf people who use sign language as their first or preferred language
Deaf community	Group of people who are culturally Deaf, who use sign language as their first or preferred language, often have a positive identity and pride attached to deafness
Deaf culture	See Deaf community
Deaf World	See Deaf community
Deafened	Used by people who have lost their hearing. Often refers to a profound level of deafness. Deafened people align themselves with the Hearing World and usually use speech rather than sign language
ENT	Hospital clinic which involves the Ear, Nose and Throat
Ependymoma	Cerebral tumour associated with NF2
Glioma	General term used for tumours of the nervous system, but can also refer to tumours arising from non-nervous cells but still in the nervous system. Often associated with NF2
GP	Family doctor
Hard of hearing	Someone with hearing loss who uses spoken language to communicate and usually has a mild-moderate loss. May be used by people with elderly-onset hearing loss

Hearing World	Mainstream hearing society. Used when comparisons are being made to the Deaf World
Meningioma	A tumour which can occur in the brain or spinal chord, often associated with NF2
NF2	Neurofibromatosis Type 2, a genetic condition that causes deafness due to tumours on the auditory nerve
NHS	National Health Service in the UK
NRCPD	National Registers of Communication Professionals Working with Deaf and Deafblind People; a group that interpreters in England, Wales and Northern Ireland should be registered with
NSL	National Sign Language (e.g. British Sign Language), with different grammar and sentence construction to spoken language
RNID	Royal National Institute for Deaf and Hard of Hearing People, UK charity
RP	Retinitis pigmentosa, visual impairment associated with Usher syndrome
Schwannoma	Benign tumour of the nerve cells, usually found in people with NF2
SSE	Sign Supported English, direct translation of spoken English

SSSL	Sign Supported Spoken Language, direct translation of spoken language
Vestibular	As in 'vestibular Schwannoma' – benign tumour on the nerve in the brain which carries information about balance and movement from the inner ear to the brain
WFD	World Federation of the Deaf

FOREWORD

This book arose out of the activities of a working party on the 'Psychosocial aspects of genetic hearing impairment', which was part of the European Union's GENDEAF project. The main aim of the group was to provide an interface between the 'hard science' of molecular and clinical geneticists on one hand and interested professionals, non-governmental organisations and the general public, on the other.

The main findings of the working party have been published in two books, '*The Impact of Genetic Hearing Impairment*' and '*The Effects of Genetic Hearing Impairment in the Family*', edited by myself and Lesley Jones (Stephens and Jones 2005, 2006). The first of these books was essentially a literature review which highlighted how little was actually known about the psychosocial aspects of genetic hearing loss and deafness. In the second, we published a number of studies which attempted to address this deficit. In addition, it also included further studies on the communication of genetic findings with members of the Deaf community, as well as with a number of different ethnic groups. However, it also highlighted the amount of further work which was needed on these topics.

The present book represents an attempt to draw together the information published in this field in a way relevant to those working with people with a range of hearing limitations. This has the aim of facilitating the lives of those with such genetic disorders by improving the understanding by professionals, in a range of medical and related disciplines, who work with them.

The three present authors have been major contributors to studies in this field. Anna Middleton has been concerned particularly with genetic understanding, communication and elucidating the views of different communities from the hard of hearing to the Deaf. Kerstin Möller has worked on many different aspects of the problems of people with deafblindness as well as with the World Health Organization's 'International Classification of Functioning, Disabilities and Health (ICF)'. Wanda Neary has written extensively on neurofibromatosis 2 (NF2), a genetic disorder resulting in total deafness as well as a number of other neurological impairments.

In this book they clearly summarise the most important elements of their knowledge in a way understandable to people with genetic hearing impairments and to the professionals who they may encounter when seeking help.

Professor Dafydd Stephens
Honorary Professor of Audiological Medicine
School of Medicine, Cardiff University, UK

PRE-PUBLICATION PEER REVIEWS

'This is a brilliant book that every health professional should read as part of their ongoing training. It is amazingly readable and gives insight into what it is like to be deaf, or deafblind. I've worked for 17 years with Deaf people and for the first time health professionals have a book that gives them sensible practical advice on working with deaf, Deaf and deafblind people.'.

Steve Powell
CEO, SignHealth, UK

'This book presents some excellent material in a wide and complex field, written with such clarity that it will be useful to almost any reader whatever their background. It will be of particular value to professionals whose work brings them into contact with people who have hearing loss, enhancing the effectiveness of their work through ensuring that they can relate well to their clients/patients. However, it will also be of interest to readers who themselves live with hearing loss, helping them understand the perspectives of the professionals they encounter.'

Dr Lorraine Gailey
CEO, Hearing Concern LINK, UK

'This is a must-read book for all health professionals. As health provision becomes increasingly the responsibility of individual patients making choices about their own care and treatment, professionals working in health not only need medical expertise but also skills in communication and information giving. For deaf and hard of hearing patients, this requires skills not often used by the average health professional; this book guides you through the maze of how to understand and communicate with a wide range of deaf and hard of hearing patients.

Well worth keeping for those times when you may be confronted by a patient that requires different communication tactics that you have never used before, and also for patients from other countries as you learn some of the useful tips of interacting with patients that communicate differently.'

Paul Redfern
Consultant: Disability & Diversity, UK

'Healthcare providers in a majority hearing/sighted society, the majority of who are themselves hearing and sighted, are likely to be unfamiliar with best practice when communicating with deaf or deafblind people, unless they are working in a speciality such as audiology. This book is a handy distillation of practical improvements that can be made in a consultation setting, many of which can be achieved by increasing one's self-awareness of the perspective of the person attending. The editor, Anna Middleton, has a professional background as a genetic counsellor and therefore a good understanding, both clinically and from a research perspective, of how clinical genetics is a particularly sensitive area of medicine for many d/Deaf people. As a result, this book may be of particular interest to clinical geneticists and genetic counsellors.'

Rachel Belk
Registered Genetic Counsellor
St Mary's Hospital, Manchester, UK

'This is an extremely useful manual for health professionals who interact with deaf and deafblind people in a clinical setting. There are sections outlining different types of hearing loss and deafness, various methods of communications and types of communicators preferred by deaf people, as well as the historical context of genetics and eugenics with respect to deafness. For those who have little experience of meeting deaf people, the case studies emphasise common pitfalls in communication, and I will be recommending the book to trainees who are new to the field.'

Dr Maria Bitner-Glindzicz
Reader in Clinical and Molecular Genetics,
UCL Institute of Child Health, and
Great Ormond Street Hospital, London, UK

'This is a new, unusual and very exciting book aimed at all health professionals. The book can serve both professionals in training but also as a guideline into a world unknown for many of us. The book is clearly structured and has a holistic approach including many components of ICF. I have worked with patients with deafblindness and NF2 for over 23 years, and I realise now that this is the first book which has addressed the basic knowledge of how to interact with people who are Deaf or Deafblind. I sincerely recommend this book.'

Prof Claes Möller
Head of Department of Audiology and Medical
Disability Research
University Hospital Örebro, Sweden

PREFACE
Anna Middleton

Use of the book

This book offers practical guidance for any health professional working with clients who have deafness or hearing loss. Such clients include those who are deaf, hard of hearing, hearing impaired, deafened, culturally Deaf, deafblind or have deafness due to neurofibromatosis type 2 (NF2).

> The work considers general communication issues relevant to both deaf sign language users and hard of hearing speech users. Specific attention is also given to the particular difficulties that sign language users face when interacting with health services.

The World Federation of the Deaf estimates there could be 70 million people with deafness across the world (WFD 2009). In the UK alone there are thought to be approximately 9 million people affected by hearing loss or deafness, which equates to 1 in 7 of the population (RNID 2008). This means that health professionals working regularly with the public will more than likely meet clients with some level of hearing loss on a daily basis.

This book is intended for use as a general reference manual to help health professionals converse effectively, for example, when a deafblind client attends an Accident and Emergency department, a Deaf client who uses sign language attends a GP surgery or a person with NF2 attends an ENT clinic. Practical advice is offered on how to prepare for the consultation, what issues need to be considered with respect to language and communication, and what cultural attitudes (relevant in a Deaf sense) may impact on the consultation.

> The intention is to provide practical information and a code of 'best practice' to help health professionals unfamiliar with deafness and hearing loss to interact effectively with others who have a variety of needs linked to deafness.

The book builds on work already published by the authors elsewhere (Middleton 2006, Neary, Stephens et al. 2006, Möller 2008). Whilst there is specific reference to working in the UK and also in Sweden, we hope that the reader will be able to apply the recommendations to their own work setting, whatever country they are from.

In September 2008 a national workshop was organised by the editor in Cardiff, UK entitled: 'Deafness and genetics: what do deaf people want?' (Middleton, Emery et al. 2008). This offered a forum for deaf and hard of hearing people from the UK to meet and mix with genetics professionals, other health professionals and academics working in the deafness field. Discussion took place around various issues surrounding clinical service provision for individuals with hearing loss and deafness in the UK. One of the outcomes of this meeting was to validate a set of recommendations for health professionals that are given in this book.

> This text is relevant to all health professionals, irrespective of their discipline or specialist area of work. It is also used as a platform for providing specific information relevant to health professionals working in Clinical Genetics departments.

Currently, genetic counselling is a service that is rarely accessed by deaf and hard of hearing clients and therefore there is a general unfamiliarity amongst geneticists and genetic counsellors about how to communicate effectively with this client group. There are specific historical sensitivities surrounding eugenics and deafness which make it particularly important that communication problems are addressed. This is relevant not only to health professionals working in Clinical Genetics but also to any other health professional who might make a referral for genetic counselling.

We do not include too much detail about diagnostic or prognostic clinical information in relation to deafness other than a brief overview, as the focus of this text is on communication. We have chosen to focus on three clinical areas only – non-syndromal deafness (i.e. deafness on its own), deafness as part of neurofibromatosis Type 2 and deafblindness. The reason these three conditions have been chosen is because they can be used as clear examples of some of the different ways that deafness can manifest and the different styles of communication that are necessary for health professionals to adopt. Many of the communication recommendations that we offer may be relevant for clients with other types of syndromal deafness.

The World Health Organization has adopted the International Classification of Functioning, Disability and Health (ICF) for classifying deafness. Here, there are two terms which are used:

- Hearing impairment refers to complete or partial loss of the ability to hear from one or both ears. The level of impairment can be mild, moderate, severe or profound
- Deafness refers to the complete loss of ability to hear from one or both ears

(World Health Organization 2001, 2006)

However, for ease of language and also to fit in with the terms deaf and hard of hearing people themselves use to describe their own deafness or hearing loss, we use the term 'deaf' or 'deaf and hard of hearing' rather than 'hearing impaired' through the majority of this book. We acknowledge that this approach may not be considered 'technically accurate' in terms of the ICF classifications. However, particularly in the UK, deaf and hard of hearing people themselves (as opposed to academics and health professionals who aim to implement the ICF definitions) are generally moving away from using the term 'hearing impaired'.

> We use the term 'deaf' as a general descriptor to refer to people with any audiological level of deafness or hearing loss, any perception of deafness and who may use either or both signed language and spoken language. Other texts use the phrases 'deaf/hard of hearing', 'hearing impaired', 'deaf/deafened/hoh', 'D/deaf' or 'people with a hearing loss' as general descriptors and our term 'deaf' should be interpreted as including all of these groups.
>
> Therefore, in this book, the word 'deaf' is used inclusively and covers people who refer to themselves as Deaf, hard of hearing or deafened.
>
> However, we also use the term 'hard of hearing' when we want to refer exclusively to speech users.
>
> The term 'hard of hearing' is also used in a generic manner to include people who call themselves 'deafened'.

We also use the collective term National Sign Language to refer to British Sign Language, American Sign Language and any other indigenous signed language used by deaf people. In contrast, the term Signed Supported Spoken Language (SSSL) refers to the literal translation of spoken language, such as Signed Supported English (SSE) in the UK. We recognise that different countries have their own equivalents to these terms.

Anti-discrimination legislation

There is legislation in different countries which aims to prevent discrimination against deaf people. In the UK, the Disability Discrimination Act (DDA) (1995) prevents deaf people from being discriminated against by any service providers, including the Health Service and hospitals (RNID 2004a). The Act expects deaf and hard of hearing people to be treated equally to their hearing counterparts. This means that every healthcare setting has a legal responsibility to ensure that communication issues are addressed and an appropriate clinical environment is provided for deaf and hard of hearing clients.

The Royal National Institute for Deaf People (RNID) in the UK has a charter called 'Louder than Words' which provides guidance for organisations to help them meet the requirements of the DDA (see www.rnid.org.uk). This offers organisations advice on how to improve their access for deaf people, from looking at door entry, reception areas, lighting, seating, policies, recruitment practices and so on. The Charter is recognised by the deaf and hard of hearing communities as a kite-mark of best practice and enables and supports organisations in complying with the DDA. The British Deaf Association (BDA), which is also called the SignCommunity, also have a BSL Charter, which aims to promote the recognition of sign language (www.bda.org.uk).

An example of potential discrimination in the clinic setting is not knowing how to take a call via a telephone relay service that enables communication through an operator (e.g. Text Relay in the UK). Another is omitting to organise an interpreter for a medical consultation and expecting the deaf client simply to lip-read the doctor; this too would be in breach of the legislation. A final example could be that of a deaf client attending a consultation accompanied by a Hearing Dog for Deaf People, but where the dog was not allowed into the clinic.

Within the UK, the law states in the Disability Discrimination Act (1995) that organisations and service providers should be proactive in making their service 'deaf friendly' rather than reactive and only responding when they have their first deaf or hard of hearing client. This book aims to offer guidance to help health service planners comply with the anti-discrimination legislation.

Work by hearing people 'on' deaf people

The vast majority of research done on deafness throughout history has been by hearing people. Many researchers, academics and health professionals have the preconceived idea that the 'poor deaf person' needs help and support to overcome their 'disability'. Nowadays it is more usual for deaf and hard of hearing people themselves to lead, organise and create their own research on deafness. There has also been a more recent insistence from funders of research to involve the consumer group that the research is aimed at, in the delivery, construction and dissemination of the findings. The editor's own research on deafness has involved a multi-skilled research team, including health professionals, academics and lay people who are deaf or hard of hearing and who use speech and/or signed language.

We are very mindful of the context within which this is written and have created this work with an open mind and an open perspective. Whilst we all happen, by coincidence, to be hearing we have worked extensively with deaf, hard of hearing and deafblind families and individuals over a number of years. We have deaf, hard of hearing and deafblind friends and colleagues; we have endeavoured to ensure that this work is relevant, appropriate and most of all not inadvertently patronising.

Acknowledgements

There have been several people and also texts that have been very influential in guiding practice and influencing research that was completed for this book. In 1995, Jamie Israel, a genetic counsellor from Gallaudet University, Washington DC, wrote the first manual for genetic counsellors on working with deaf people and families (Israel 1995). Despite its age, this work is still very current and offers a thorough account, together with practical advice on how to best serve deaf clients. We hope we have been able to build on this seminal text. Also recognition goes to Kathleen Arnos, Gallaudet University, who was one of the first people to publish work on how genetics services for deaf people should be structured (Arnos, Israel et al. 1991, 1992).

Particular recognition goes to Dafydd Stephens from the School of Medicine, Cardiff University, the leader of the GENDEAF European Union Thematic Network Project (2001–2005) subgroup on psychosocial aspects of genetics and deafness. Dafydd had the vision and expertise to bring together health professionals, researchers and academics interested in psychosocial issues and deafness. He was particularly influential in enabling this book to be written.

This book is published with the support of the European Commission, Fifth Framework programme, Quality of Life and Management of Living Resources programme. It does not represent the opinion of the European Community and the European Community is not responsible for any use that might be made of the data appearing herein.

Enormous thanks go to Steve Powell, Rachel Belk, Cathy Middleton, Dafydd Stephens, Lorraine Gailey,

Maria Bitner-Glindzicz, Claes Möller and Paul Redfern for reviewing the content of this book prior to publication.

The authors

The authors all belonged to the GENDEAF European Union Thematic Network Project (2001–2005), and it is through this that the idea for the book was developed.

Work done by the editor as part of a Health Services Research, Department of Health funded research project (2005–2009) entitled 'deaf individuals' understanding and perception of genetics and their needs from a genetic counselling service' has been very influential in guiding the content of this book. Many of the recommendations for deaf clients are based on research evidence gathered in the Department of Health project.

Anna Middleton is a Consultant Research Genetic Counsellor and Registered Genetic Counsellor working at the School of Medicine, Cardiff University. She has been working as a genetic counsellor since 1995 and completed her PhD in 1999; this involved gathering the attitudes of deaf and hard of hearing people towards prenatal testing for inherited deafness. Anna has written extensively on the attitudes that deaf and hard of hearing people have towards various issues surrounding genetics. The years 2005–2009 were spent running a national research project which involved interviewing Deaf people in sign language to gather their views about genetics, genetic counselling, access to the health service and communication issues. This research also ascertained attitudes towards using health services, collected via a specially designed written questionnaire for deaf, deafened and hard of hearing people. Anna has worked clinically within the NHS as a general genetic counsellor at St James's Hospital in Leeds and as a specialist cancer genetic counsellor at Addenbrooke's Hospital in Cambridge. Between the years 2004 and 2010 Anna was Vice-Chair of the Genetic Counsellor Registration Board in the UK and in this role has written policy and guidelines for the UK genetic counselling profession. Anna has worked for Homerton College at the University of Cambridge as an associate lecturer on genetic counselling and has also taught on the two UK MSc Genetic Counselling courses in Manchester and Cardiff. Since 1999 she has also been the UK representative on the editorial board of the Journal of Genetic Counselling.

Wanda Neary is a Consultant Community Paediatrician (Paediatric Audiology), working in Warrington Community Services Unit. She has been involved in collaborative research with the Department of Otolaryngology Head and Neck Surgery, Manchester Royal Infirmary, the Department of Medical Genetics, St Mary's Hospital Manchester, and the Welsh Hearing Institute, Cardiff. Her special research interest from 1989 has been in the field of neurofibromatosis Type 2 (NF2).

Kerstin Möller has an MSc in Management of Health and Welfare Organisations, and a PhD in Disability Research.

She has conducted public investigations of services for people with deafblindness on behalf of the Swedish Ministry of Social Affairs and the Swedish National Agency for Education. She has done consultancy for the Nordic Staff Training Centre for Deafblind Services, the Swedish Resource Centre for Matters regarding Deafblindness and the Swedish Association of Rare Disorders. She teaches students, professionals and people with deafblindness and their next of kin in deafblindness know-how. She works as a supervisor at Research & Development in Sörmland and is associated to the Swedish Institute of Disability Research including HEAD and Audiological Research Centre at Örebro University Hospital.

Chapter 1

Facts and figures about deafness, NF2 and deafblindness

Anna Middleton, Wanda Neary
and Kerstin Möller

Overview of deafness and hearing loss

The clinical impact of deafness is variable. It may occur at any stage of life, it may impact on the individual's ability to function on a day-to-day basis and it may or may not be disabling.

Conversational speech can be measured as having a loudness of approximately 60 decibels (dB). Hearing is considered significantly restricted when the ear cannot interpret or process sounds of 25 dB or more.

The following is adapted from work by Prosser and Martini (2007).

- An individual with a '**mild**' hearing loss can only begin to hear sound if it is between 20 and 40 dB. They may have difficulty understanding conversations in a noisy room, or if the speaker is far away, but should be able to hear one-to-one conversations if the speaker's voice is not too soft. They may have problems hearing a person in front of them who is whispering.

Working with Deaf People – a Handbook for Health Professionals, ed. Anna Middleton. Published by Cambridge University Press.

- An individual with a '**moderate**' hearing loss can begin to hear sound between 41 and 70 dB; people with such a loss have difficulty understanding normal conversational levels of speech, but may be able to hear loud noises, for example the sound of a lawnmower (about 90 dB).
- An individual with a '**severe**' hearing loss begins to hear sound between 71 and 95 dB. Such people will only be able to hear an individual speaker if they are at close range and the speaker is shouting; they may be able to hear a car horn (110 dB). A person with a mild, moderate or severe hearing loss may receive benefit from the use of a hearing aid.
- An individual with a '**profound**' hearing loss can only hear sound equivalent to or over 95 dB, for example a gunshot (140 dB). Profoundly deaf people will not be able to hear loud speech or background noise and may prefer to use sign language rather than speech as their form of communication. Some profoundly deaf people may also not receive much benefit from a hearing aid and as such may choose not to wear one.

(Prosser and Martini 2007)

Terminology

There is often confusion about the terms used to describe deafness. This is largely because health professionals, academics and deaf and hard of hearing individuals themselves may use different terminology to describe related concepts (Grundfast and Rosen 1992).

- Generally speaking, clinicians and molecular deafness academics often use the term 'hearing impaired' rather than 'deaf' as this latter term is often considered too non-specific. 'Hearing impaired' has a precise medical definition, as per the International Classification of Functioning, Disability and Health (Stephens and Danermark 2005).
- However, the term 'hearing impaired' is often not viewed as politically correct these days. It tends to be avoided by deaf and hard of hearing people themselves, as they do not like to be perceived as being defective or 'impaired'.
- Use of the phrase '*the* deaf' is also not perceived as politically correct either as it has a slightly condescending air to it. This has been replaced by the use of 'deaf people' or 'people with deafness' instead. For example, in the UK the charity 'Hearing Dogs for *the* Deaf' is now termed 'Hearing Dogs for Deaf People'.
- Many people with disabilities have suggested it is most politically correct to refer to the *person* first and the 'disability' second, for example, 'people with Down's syndrome' rather than 'the Down's client'. This phraseology may only partly apply to deafness – it is still acceptable to say 'deaf people' because deafness can be tied up with identity. But for the hard of hearing group it may be considered more sensitive to use the term 'people with hearing loss'.

- Those with a mild or moderate level of deafness will often refer to themselves as being hard of hearing or having a hearing loss. Such people may also find great benefit from wearing a hearing aid and tend to use spoken language rather than signed language. Within interactions with hearing people they will often be able to use their residual hearing and amplified hearing as well as lip-reading to help their communication. People who have elderly-onset hearing loss often call themselves hard of hearing.

- People who are 'deafened' tend to have a profound level of deafness and usually will have started life as a hearing person. Their deafness may be progressive or may have a sudden onset. Deafened people usually feel they belong to the Hearing World rather than the Deaf community as they often do not use sign language. They may also receive little benefit from hearing aids, although cochlear implants may work well for this group. Within interactions with hearing people, deafened people may rely very heavily on lip-reading, writing and reading to communicate.

*d*eaf and *D*eaf

The following text provides a very general guide to the use of the terms deaf, hard of hearing, deafened and Deaf in the UK. These concepts are fluid and changeable and there are no universally accepted definitions, used by affected people themselves, that translate across the world. However, we have attempted to capture the way the terms are broadly used.

- People who refer to themselves as 'deaf' usually have a profound level of deafness, which may also be static rather than progressive.

People who refer to themselves as 'Deaf' (written with an uppercase D) are indicating that they have a culture and identity that is linked in with their deafness and that they use sign language as their preferred communication (Padden and Humphries 2005).

- Those who refer to themselves as 'deaf' may use some spoken language and some sign language in different contexts. Alternatively, they may prefer to only use sign language. They may also feel most comfortable within the Deaf World/community/culture (a minority group within mainstream society where those who belong mainly communicate in sign language).
- Some who refer to themselves as 'hard of hearing' may do so to indicate that they *are not* profoundly deaf and yet they may still mix within the Deaf community, and thus may use both sign language and spoken communication in different situations.
- Conversely some people call themselves 'hard of hearing' or 'deafened' to indicate that they are not part of the Deaf community.

People who refer to themselves as 'hard of hearing', 'hearing impaired' or 'deafened' often feel they belong to the Hearing World and/or Hard of Hearing World (consisting of other people with a similar perception of hearing loss). This tends to be a group that is not fluent in sign language and relies on using spoken language.

Case study: developing a Deaf identity

Jo from Northern Ireland had been profoundly deaf since birth, as were his mother and maternal grandfather. Jo had a severe level of deafness, together with a white forelock and different-coloured eyes. He was diagnosed by his paediatrician as having Waardenburg syndrome.

At age 5, Jo found it difficult to fit into the mainstream hearing school recommended by his Local Education Authority and so his parents decided to send him to a specialist school for deaf children, similar to the one his mother had been to. Here he was offered a Total Communication approach – and so had speech therapy to help him learn speech, but also he learnt sign language.

By the age of 10 he found mixing with other deaf children gave him a sense of normality that he didn't feel amongst hearing children and gradually he found he felt more comfortable using sign language rather than speech. Both his parents were members of the local Deaf club and also used sign language at home.

Over time Jo found that his experiences in school and at the local Deaf club helped him to develop a Deaf identity – he felt more comfortable mixing with other Deaf people and communicating in sign language. After leaving school he trained to become a social worker for deaf people.

Terms used by people with NF2

- People with NF2 are born into the Hearing World; they usually use spoken language when communicating.
- When they develop hearing loss, which is most commonly in their 20s or 30s, people with NF2 usually describe themselves as deaf.
- Most people with NF2 learn to lip-read; they use speech and written communication.
- Some receive a cochlear implant, or an auditory brainstem implant, which aids their lip-reading.
- Only a small minority of people with NF2 learn to communicate using an NSL and consider themselves part of the Deaf community.

Terms used by people with deafblindness

- People with deafblindness are a heterogeneous group. Those who are born with a hearing loss will often call themselves hearing impaired or deaf.
- As their sight deteriorates they may call themselves 'deaf with visual impairment'.

- If they have learnt sign language as their first language they may call themselves Deaf.
- Some people call themselves deafblind; however, many are not aware that the combination of their hearing and visual loss is significant and so may just mention one sensory loss.
- Using the term 'impairment' in the label 'visual impairment' is politically correct; there is not the same stigma attached to this term as there is for 'hearing impairment' for those who have deafness in isolation.
- For ease of language and reading the term 'deafness' and 'deaf people' is used collectively in this book to refer to people with any level and perception of hearing loss.

deaf
- general term for all levels of deafness
- tends to refer to profound, prelingual deafness or deafness caused by NF2
- speech and/or sign language

hard of hearing
- mild – severe level of hearing loss
- possibly progressive
- possibly postlingual
- may be elderly onset
- speech user

Deaf
- culturally Deaf
- uses sign language as preferred language

deafened
- gone deaf later in life or postlingually
- usually a profound level of deafness
- speech user

hearing impaired
- often used by health professionals
- word 'impaired' not seen as very politically correct by some
- used by people with deafblindness
- speech user

Deafness can be perceived in different ways

- A person who considers themselves hard of hearing or deafened may find their hearing loss is an irritation for them and their significant others. They may also have to make large adjustments in their life both practically and emotionally in order to adapt to this.
- A person who considers themselves culturally Deaf may feel a sense of pride in their deafness and may not feel it is a problem at all (Ladd 1988, 2003) – in fact within their family and social position, they may feel that it is preferable to be deaf rather than hearing.

Deaf sign language users and hard of hearing speech users may have completely opposing views and perspectives towards deafness.

Having a clear family history of deafness can be very positive for individuals who are deaf. Several research studies have shown that, irrespective of the level of deafness, age of onset or impact of deafness, if there are other relatives who can be role models for the individual who is deaf, then this can be of enormous psychological benefit (Stephens 2007).

Frequency of deafness, NF2 and deafblindness

- In the developed world deafness is the most common congenital disorder (Hilgert, Smith et al. 2008).

- Approximately 1 in 500 babies are born with a hearing loss greater than 40 dB (Morton and Nance 2006).
- Hearing loss increases with age; 16% of adults have a bilateral hearing loss greater than 25 dB (Davis 1989, Morton 1991) and by the age of 80 nearly half the population will have a hearing loss greater than 25 dB (Morton 1991).
- The diagnostic prevalence of NF2 is 1 in 210,000 and the birth incidence has been estimated to be approximately 1 in 40,000 (Evans, Huson et al. 1992a); many individuals do not develop features of the condition until the third decade or later, although individuals with aggressive disease die before the third decade.
- The vast majority of people with NF2 develop deafness either due to the presence of vestibular Schwannomas (tumours of the eighth nerve) or due to the surgical removal of vestibular Schwannomas.
- Deafblindness is very rare, especially in young people. Prelingual deafblindness affects 1 in 10,000 children (Möller 2007).
- Usher syndrome affects about 3 per 100,000 (Sadeghi 2005).
- Developing a combination of visual and hearing impairment increases with age and particularly after the 7th decade.
- Visual impairment is the most common impairment in people with hearing loss. Thirty per cent of children with hearing loss or deafness have been found to have visual impairment (Nikolopoulos, Lioumi et al. 2006).

Describing deafness and hearing loss

A variety of different categories are used by health professionals to describe deafness. Classification can be made in different ways dependent on the cause, the form and the stage of life at which it occurred:

Type of deafness:	sensorineural vs. conductive
Timing of deafness:	congenital vs. acquired
	prelingual vs. postlingual
	late vs. early onset
Progression of deafness:	progressive vs. non-progressive
Cause of deafness:	genetic vs. environmental
Form of deafness:	syndromal vs. non-syndromal

A brief discussion of each of these follows.

Sensorineural vs. conductive deafness

When the structures within the inner ear or auditory nerve are changed or missing, for example, involving the cochlear hair cells, the result is *sensorineural* deafness, whereas structural changes in the outer and middle ear result in *conductive* deafness. A mixture of sensorineural and conductive factors leads to *mixed* deafness.

Congenital vs. acquired

Congenital means that a person has been born deaf whereas *acquired* means that a person has become deaf as a result of environmental factors, for instance noise or industrial damage or infection. Congenital deafness is mostly sensorineural in origin. Deafness occurring in older age is sometimes referred to as 'an acquired sensorineural' form of deafness.

Prelingual vs. postlingual

Prelingual means that deafness existed before the development of language skills. This term is sometimes used interchangeably with the term *congenital.* If deafness occurs after the development of language skills this is described as *postlingual.*

Early vs. late onset

Early onset and *late onset* refer to the time when the deafness occurred, i.e. in childhood or adulthood.

Progressive vs. non-progressive

Progressive refers to the increasing severity of the condition over time, whereas *non-progressive* means that the severity has not changed over time and remains fairly consistent.

Genetic vs. environmental

Babies born with severe-profound, congenital or early-onset deafness have their deafness due to genetic causes in > 50% of cases, whereas environmental causes are believed to account for < 50% of cases, with the remainder being of unknown cause (Parving 1983, 1984, Newton 1985).

Syndromal vs. non-syndromal

One-third of all cases of genetic deafness are *syndromal*; *non-syndromal* deafness accounts for the other two-thirds (Reardon and Pembrey 1990). Syndromal deafness includes other clinical features, for example blindness, craniofacial defects and pigmentation problems. The most common of these are Waardenburg syndrome, Usher syndrome, Pendred syndrome, CHARGE, neurofibromatosis Type II and branchio-oto-renal syndrome. Deafness is involved in over 400 genetic syndromes (Toriello, Reardon et al. 2004).

At least 20 different genetic syndromes are associated with prelingual deafblindness (Möller 2007). More than 50 hereditary syndromes are known to cause acquired deafblindness (Möller 2007).

When genetic deafness occurs in isolation with no other clinical features, it is known as *non-syndromal* deafness. There are over 50 non-syndromal deafness genes where alterations (mutations) have been identified. It is therefore technically possible to offer genetic testing for these genes, but testing may not be available clinically (Smith and Van Camp 2008).

Causes of deafness

There are many different causes of deafness; these include environmental and genetic factors.

- More than half of congenital or prelingual deafness has a genetic cause (Smith and Van Camp 2008).
- Several hundred genes are known to be involved with deafness (Smith and Van Camp 2008).
- Approximately 50% of non-syndromal prelingual deafness, with a genetic basis, is caused by alterations in the GJB2 and GJB6 genes. Approximately 1 in 50 people are carriers of the alterations in the GJB2 gene (Estivill, Fortina et al. 1998, Kelley, Harris et al. 1998, Smith and Van Camp 2008).
- Late-onset or 'elderly' hearing loss has always been thought to be due to environmental causes, but more recently it has been discovered that this has a probable genetic basis. This basis is still being investigated (Smith and Van Camp 2008).
- The most frequent environmental cause of congenital deafness is infection with cytomegalovirus (CMV) (Smith and Van Camp 2008).
- People who call themselves 'deafened' may be deaf due to a number of different reasons; for example, meningitis, head injury, otosclerosis, viral infections and ototoxic medications.

Case study: moderate hearing loss, use of speech

Jane was born to a hearing family in Wales – her parents, grandparents and siblings were all hearing. So, when she was diagnosed as having a moderate level of deafness by the Newborn Hearing Screening project, this was a great shock to the family.

Jane had congenital, bilateral, sensorineural deafness and was fitted with hearing aids. Jane's parents decided that they wanted to raise her within the wider hearing society and so with the help of a teacher for deaf children and additional speech therapy support at home Jane learnt to lip-read and use speech.

Jane's parents had genetic counselling in order to determine whether there was a genetic basis to Jane's deafness. Genetic testing revealed that Jane had inherited two alterations in the GJB2 gene, one from each of her parents, who carried these. Parents who are both carriers for these gene alterations have a 1 in 4 or 25% chance of having deaf children.

Comment

The GJB2 or Connexin 26 gene is the most common gene causing deafness. It mainly results in a child being born with deafness for the first time in a hearing family, where both parents of the child with deafness are hearing but carry an alteration in the gene.

Neurofibromatosis Type 2 (NF2)

- NF2 is a syndrome which usually results in total deafness. It is characterised by the presence of bilateral vestibular Schwannomas of the eighth nerve (benign tumours of the hearing nerve on both sides).
- Other tumours of the central and peripheral nervous system, such as meningiomas, gliomas, ependymomas and peripheral Schwannomas, are associated with NF2.
- NF2 is a dominantly inherited genetic condition caused by a defect on chromosome 22.
- There is a family history of NF2 in 50% of cases, but in the remaining 50% the condition arises as a result of a new genetic change.
- There is an aggressive form of the condition with an early onset, the presence of multiple nervous system tumours and premature death.
- In some individuals who are affected only with bilateral eighth-nerve tumours, the condition may progress slowly and they may retain their hearing into their seventh decade.
- NF2 is a clinically and genetically different condition from neurofibromatosis Type 1, which is a much more common genetic condition.

Presenting symptoms of NF2

- The majority of adult individuals with NF2 present with unilateral hearing loss, tinnitus, imbalance and vertigo, related to the presence of bilateral vestibular Schwannomas. Bilateral vestibular Schwannomas are usually present at diagnosis though only one may initially be causing hearing loss.

- The mean age at onset of symptoms is in the second and third decades.
- Two types of NF2 can be recognised – Wishart and Gardner.
- The Wishart type presents at an early age, the disease progression is rapid, and the individual has multiple other tumours of the central and peripheral nervous system in addition to bilateral vestibular Schwannomas.
- The onset of the Gardner type is at a later age and it has a more benign course with bilateral vestibular Schwannomas but no other tumours of the nervous system.
- Children aged 10 years or younger who are diagnosed with NF2 (a relatively rare occurrence) frequently present with symptoms of an isolated tumour of the nervous system rather than with symptoms due to bilateral vestibular Schwannomas (Evans, Birch et al. 1999).
- The diagnostic criteria for NF2 are given in the Appendix.

Diagnosis

- An MRI scan of the head and spine is the gold standard in diagnostic terms, with the possibility of revealing tumours as small as 2 to 3 mm in size.

- Presymptomatic DNA diagnosis of NF2 can be undertaken using molecular genetic techniques.

Case study: a new diagnosis of NF2

Tariq is a young man of 17 years. He has noted increasing difficulty with his left-sided hearing over a period of 12 months, and is now unable to hear a telephone conversation with his left ear. During the last 3 months he has also been troubled with continuous high-pitched left-sided tinnitus. There is no family history of deafness. His doctor refers him to the local ENT clinic, where the presence of a left-sided sensorineural hearing loss is confirmed. An MRI scan indicates bilateral vestibular Schwannomas, left greater than right. Tariq is referred to a specialist multidisciplinary NF2 clinic for further management.

Tariq is shocked at the diagnosis, and has many questions to put to the specialist multidisciplinary team regarding the impact of NF2 on his future career, his personal relationships and his general health. Further management of his eighth-nerve tumours is in the hands of the neuro-otologist and neurosurgeon. The geneticist explains the implications for Tariq's future children. Tariq is introduced to an NF2 support worker.

Comment

Members of the specialist multidisciplinary team must be sensitive to the psychological impact of NF2 as a potentially life-changing disease for Tariq and his family. The situation is particularly difficult as there is no family history of NF2, and Tariq's illness has presented for the first time. The prospect of total eventual hearing loss and change in Tariq's plans for future employment may be devastating. Parental anxieties and possible feelings of guilt may be considerable. Members of the multidisciplinary team must ensure, as much as possible, that Tariq is prepared for the psychological blow of eventual total hearing loss and initiate appropriate training in non-auditory communication skills.

Management and treatment of NF2

NF2 presents marked challenges to clinicians with regard to the diagnosis as well as medical and surgical treatment (Neary, Stephens et al. 2006). Members of the affected person's family require screening for the condition, together with genetic counselling. The specialist role of regional and national centres with multidisciplinary teams involved in the management of all aspects of NF2 has been emphasised (Evans, Baser et al. 2005).

Clinicians need to be sensitive to the potentially life-changing psychological impact of the diagnosis of NF2, with the knowledge of eventual total hearing loss in the affected person (Neary, Stephens et al. 2006).

In families where the condition has appeared for the first time, the impact is even more marked. The prospect of future total deafness faces a person who on the surface appears healthy, and may have presented with only a mild hearing loss. Feelings of guilt and anxiety are common at this stage. A treatment strategy needs to be formulated which conserves useful hearing and aims for a good quality of life without causing complications that involve the facial nerve or neurological status. Training in lip-reading as well as other communication methods needs to be implemented as soon as possible.

The eighth nerve is very close to the facial nerves and so when vestibular Schwannomas are surgically removed, even by very skilled surgeons, it is possible to damage the facial nerve in this process. Minimising surgical damage to the facial nerve is paramount as bilateral facial weakness may result in physical difficulties relating to eating and smiling etc. and is often cosmetically distressing to the client. In NF2, the eyes may become affected, for example through damage to tear production as well as the blink reflex.

The primary goal of management is to foresee and take steps to avoid life-threatening events. The affected individual should be reviewed by the specialist team on a regular basis, when MRI of the neural axis should be undertaken. In this way impending complications should be identified and the need for surgery indicated in a timely manner.

When both auditory nerves are affected and the client with NF2 is totally deaf, an auditory brainstem implant

(ABI) is usually inserted. The ABI is reported to enhance lip-reading skills as well as providing an awareness of environmental sound, although the ABI usually does not result in good levels of hearing.

Deafblindness

In everyday terms, deaf and blind denote individual impairments and deafblind denotes a combination of the two impairments. People who have complete loss of both vision and hearing are very rare. Six per cent of those regarded as having deafblindness were found to have total visual and hearing impairment (Wolf-Schein 1989). Thus denoting deafblindness solely by total visual impairment (blindness) and total hearing impairment (deafness) is, in general, used neither by professionals in the field nor by organisations for people with combined visual and hearing impairment. There is no consensus definition of deafblindness.

In the USA, at the Helen Keller National Center for Youths and Adults who are Deaf-Blind (HKNC), deafblindness is defined as the degree of visual function and degree of hearing function. Historically, the primary education system in Sweden has referred to children with deafblindness as 'three-sensed' (Liljedahl 1993), which emphasises the senses left. In 2007, the Nordic Staff Training Centre adopted a new Nordic definition for the Deafblind Service which highlights special requirements rather than the degree of the two impairments.

> 'Deafblindness is a distinct disability. Deafblindness is a combined vision and hearing disability. It limits activities of a person and restricts full participation in society to such a degree that society is required to facilitate specific services, environmental alterations and/or technology' (www.nud.dk).

Finally, there is the classification based on International Classification of Functioning, Disability and Health (ICF) that combines the degree of sensory impairment, activity limitations and participation restrictions with environmental factors. The fact that visible and audible signals are not processed normally is an impairment of body function. Thus seeing/watching and hearing/listening activities become limited and the visible and audible information cannot be interpreted in an intelligible way (Möller 2008).

> Based on self-reports within deaf studies, deafblindness is regarded to be an alternative way of perceiving the world, though often as an 'isolated island' (Barnett 2002c). Reports from people with deafblindness show strategies and habits used for 'negotiating a place in a hostile world' (Schneider 2006).

Heterogeneity of the group

The population is distributed across all ages, with onset of one or both impairments at different ages. Some people first develop hearing impairment, others vice versa, while a few develop severe to profound visual and hearing impairment at the same time.

The group is often subdivided according to the age of the observed onset. In *prelingual onset,* the impact of both impairments comes before or during the development of language skills. Professionals usually call this subgroup congenital deafblindness. *Postlingual onset* is often called acquired deafblindness. The third group is *elderly* people who develop combined visual and hearing impairment at an old age.

Some conditions which cause deafblindness

The rarity of these conditions and difficulties in assessment increase the risk of an incorrect diagnosis, which also may be 'hidden' due to other dysfunctions and thus attributed to other conditions (McInnes and Treffry 1982, Möller 2007).

Usher syndrome

- Usher syndrome (USH) is a genetic disorder with autosomal recessive inheritance.
- USH is the most common cause of deafblindness before old age (Kimberling and Möller 1995, Sadeghi 2005). The

syndrome is divided into three distinct clinical types (types I–III). Different gene mutations and clinical features distinguish these types.

- USH affects the structure of the cochlea, the vestibular organ (types I and III) and the retina bilaterally (Kimberling and Möller 1995).
- In the inner ear (cochlea and the labyrinth) the hair cells are affected.
- The disorder in the eye, retinitis pigmentosa (RP), is one of several genetic disorders affecting the retina (Hartong, Berson et al. 2006). The visual deterioration is slower in USH compared to some other forms of RP (Sadeghi 2005).

USH type I is associated with profound deafness, while types II and III are associated with moderate to severe hearing impairment. In type III this is usually progressive (Kimberling and Möller 1995, Sadeghi 2005).

- Vestibular function is absent bilaterally in USH type I. This will result in a delayed walking age (>18 months) and clumsiness, especially in dimly lit situations or in darkness (Möller 2007).
- Type II has normal vestibular function, while type III has progressive loss of vestibular function.
- All three types of USH cause progressive visual impairment (Kimberling and Möller 1995).

- The RP in the three types of USH does not differ as much as the auditory or vestibular functions. In many cases the progression of visual impairment can be the same in types I, II and III.

Rehabilitation of children with USH type 1 has changed dramatically with the introduction of cochlear implants (CIs). Children with USH type 1 in Sweden are fitted with two implants at the age of 6–12 months. The aim is for them to hear spoken language and to develop speech. From around 1997, nearly 95% of all children with congenital profound deafness (including USH type 1) have received cochlear implants (Möller 2007). 'Treating' deafness when it occurs in conjunction with blindness tends to be approached from a medical model; however, this is not always the case. There are still some people with Usher syndrome who prefer to view their deafness from the cultural model and would prefer not to have a treatment such as a cochlear implant.

Alström syndrome

- Alström syndrome is a hereditary autosomal recessive disorder.
- All individuals with the disease have visual impairment, hearing loss, obesity problems, cardiovascular problems, early-onset diabetes type 2 and susceptibility to infection. Other organs such as kidneys, pancreas and liver can also be affected.

- An early symptom in infancy is light sensitivity.
- Vision problems due to RP will decline rapidly, although the degree of visual impairment varies. The vast majority of young adults with Alström will be blind by the age of 14 years.
- At the age of 4–6 years hearing loss is evident in most children with Alström syndrome.
- Over 500 cases of Alström syndrome are known worldwide.
- This is a condition causing gradual degeneration of the retina. As a result, the eye gradually loses its ability to capture and process light, night vision decreases and the child experiences loss of peripheral vision.
- An early sign of loss of vision may be that the child trips often and has trouble finding things. Vision will decline rapidly, although the degree of visual impairment varies.

Charge

- This is a syndrome that is autosomal dominant.
- The name is derived from the first letter of the organs that are most often affected. **C** stands for **c**oloboma (defect in the development of the eye), **H** for **h**eart defect, **A** for **a**tresia choane (narrowing of the opening between the nasal cavity and the pharynx), **R** for **r**etardation of growth and/or development, **G** for **g**enital anomalies and **E** represents **e**ar anomalies with or without hearing loss.

- The incidence is around 1 in 12,000 (Firth and Hurst 2005).
- Malformation of the outer and middle ear is common; malformation of the bones of the middle ear results in a conductive hearing loss.
- A malformed cochlea occurs in 90%. Small or absent semicircular canals cause sensorineural hearing loss and balance impairment.
- Many children with CHARGE have severe problems with breathing, swallowing or speech, and some have severe learning difficulties.

Congenital rubella syndrome (CRS)

- CRS is also known as German measles.
- Pregnant women who become infected with rubella in the first 12 weeks of pregnancy can infect their baby with the virus.
- The classic three features of congenital rubella syndrome are deafness, blindness and heart disease, although there are other possible symptoms that can occur such as learning difficulties and developmental delay.

Older people

- Degeneration of the macula, which is associated with older age, causes central visual field loss.

- Age-related hearing loss in combination with different diseases affecting the eye is very common over the age of 65 and prevalence increases with age.

> Older people with combined visual and hearing loss comprise the largest group of people who have deafblindness.

Chapter 2

General themes to consider when working with deaf and hard of hearing clients

Anna Middleton

This chapter considers general communication issues that are relevant to deafness and hearing loss. Specific issues pertinent to people who are deaf due to NF2 and people who have deafblindness are considered in Chapters 4 and 5 respectively.

Seeing a hearing aid

- When meeting a deaf or hard of hearing person for the first time, seeing a hearing aid may offer some clues as to the form of communication the person uses.
- It is possible that they identify more with the Hearing World and if so will use lip-reading and speech to communicate.
- Alternatively they may still be culturally Deaf and prefer to use sign language, but for interactions with hearing people prefer to utilise the residual hearing they have as

Working with Deaf People – a Handbook for Health Professionals, ed. Anna Middleton. Published by Cambridge University Press. © Cambridge University Press 2010.

this helps them with lip-reading. A Deaf person may also like to wear a hearing aid as it may offer help with ambient noise; for example, in a city where there is noisy traffic, having the hearing aid switched on may help with crossing the road and knowing where the traffic is coming from.

It should not be assumed if no hearing aid is seen that a person is not deaf; it may be that they are profoundly deaf and gain limited use from a hearing aid or are culturally Deaf and may just prefer not to wear one, or it may also mean that they have an as yet undiagnosed hearing loss.

Case study: seeing no hearing aids on a sign language user

Shan lived in the UK and had been profoundly deaf from birth. She used sign language as her first language and although she had been fitted with a hearing aid when she was a child had long thrown these away as they were more of a hindrance than a help. She also found that as she preferred to use sign language the hearing aids sometimes gave the impression to people that she could hear and use speech and this annoyed her. Also, she found that people sometimes stared at her hearing aid and so this was also a reason she just preferred not to wear one.

On a routine visit to her GP Shan approached the receptionist and pointed to her ears while mouthing the word 'deaf'. She indicated that she wanted to write something down and the receptionist handed her a pen and some paper. Shan wrote 'appointment please today GP'. The receptionist understood what Shan wanted and so looked through the diary. Shan smiled and signed the word for deaf, which involves touching the ear; she then used sign language to indicate that she was a signer. The receptionist assumed Shan must be trying to tell her that she had forgotten to put her hearing aids in as she saw Shan touching her ear; the receptionist wrongly assumed all deaf people wore them. In fact, Shan just wanted to make it clear that she was a deaf sign language user.

Comments

The Department of Health in the UK recommend that all front-line health service staff receive deaf awareness training (Department of Health 2005). The receptionist was unaware that some deaf people do not wear a hearing aid. In addition to booking an appointment for Shan it would have also been helpful if she had asked about her communication needs and made arrangements so these could be met in the consultation with the GP.

Dissatisfaction with the health services

Existing healthcare services for people with deafness are known to be suboptimal (Steinberg, Sullivan et al. 1998,

Ubido, Huntington et al. 2002, Iezzoni, O'Day et al. 2004, RNID 2004b, Reeves and Kokoruwe 2005, Steinberg, Barnett et al. 2006). This has led to a depressing level of dissatisfaction from deaf people about using them. The main problems are lack of deaf awareness amongst health professionals and inappropriate provision of communication support. This has led to a distrust, apprehension and negativity from many people about interacting with health professionals.

In 2004, the Royal National Institute for Deaf People (RNID), the UK's largest deafness charity, indicated that 'urgent action' was needed to improve the accessibility and communication for deaf and hard of hearing people using the National Health Service (NHS) in the UK. They also recommended that all front-line NHS staff should have deaf awareness training (RNID 2004b). This is also recommended by the Department of Health in the UK (Department of Health 2005).

Lisa Harmer from the University of Rochester has written a useful review of research surrounding health services and deaf people (Harmer 1999). The following text is a quotation from this work and summarises very neatly some research in this area:

'A nonrandomized survey of d/hoh people by Zazove et al. (1993) reported that deaf people visit physicians more frequently than do hearing people, but the deaf individuals report less satisfaction with the health care

> services they received.... Zazove hypothesized that deaf individuals may keep returning to physicians to seek assistance for problems and answers to questions that were not understood in prior visits. In that study d/hoh individuals also said when they attempted to exchange written notes with their doctor, the doctor's writing was often illegible, or the physician wrote at a level that was beyond the literacy skills of the client. In addition, patients regularly underwent tests or received prescriptions without understanding why the action had been undertaken.' (Harmer 1999, pp. 77–8)

Very similar findings have also been reported by the Royal National Institute for Deaf People in the UK (Dye and Kyle 2001, RNID 2004b) and also in the author's own work (Middleton, Turner et al. 2009).

- There has been a consistent lack of understanding amongst health professionals about the different ways of perceiving deafness.
- There has been a consistent lack of deaf awareness in the health service. This not only applies to deaf and Deaf people but also to those who are hard of hearing or deafened.
- Many Deaf people do not want to have a cochlear implant (Harmer 1999) and resent the assumption that there is something negligent about this attitude.

Case study: struggling to communicate in Accident and Emergency

Dominic is culturally Deaf. He works for his local Deaf community and mixes regularly with other Deaf people. He had been educated at a mainstream hearing school and had dropped out of school at 15 as his special needs were not being met. He found it difficult to learn speech and communicate with his hearing peers. He developed his Deaf identity from a sense of survival, and felt that it was only other culturally Deaf people who really understood him. He was involved in the march in London to have BSL recognised as a British language and was a prominent disability rights activist.

Dominic attends the Accident and Emergency department in his local hospital because he has broken his arm in a clash with police. Because of the pain in his arm he cannot sign properly nor write. When he arrives in A+E the doctor cannot understand what he is saying and struggles to communicate; he can see that Dominic is frustrated, frightened and angry. Dominic is defensive and shouts at the doctor; what he says sounds like 'interpreter'! The A+E doctor is just finishing a very busy shift and he is tired and could do without any confrontation. He asks one of the nurses if Dominic has a cochlear implant. Dominic lip-reads the words 'cochlear implant' and is livid. He shouts at the doctor 'IGNORANT'! and begins to cry.

One of the reception staff has recently done a signing class at night school and she hears this interaction. She comes over to Dominic and signs to him, 'I'm so sorry, I can see you are really upset, my signing isn't great, but I will sort out an interpreter immediately for you'. He looks at her in disbelief, surprised that suddenly there is an open line of communication. The fear in his face gradually lessens and he signs back to her 'thank you'. He feels he can now wait for an interpreter and relaxes a little as he will soon have the opportunity to express himself clearly to the doctor.

Comments

The A+E doctor was unaware that his question about a cochlear implant would cause such a reaction in Dominic; he didn't intend to inflame an already emotional situation. Once an interpreter arrives it may be helpful for the doctor to have a chat with Dominic and to say that he didn't mean to cause offence.

Some deaf and hard of hearing people have also had such a negative experience of health services in the past that they feel very defensive. On arrival at A+E there should be staff available on every shift to set up appropriate communication aids, for example, immediate access to an on-site interpreter, or access to a live on-line interpreting

---

(*Continued*)

service,[1] or preferably a member of staff who can communicate in sign language, even if at a basic level. Dominic should not be expected to lip-read and write to communicate in this situation; **in the UK it is the hospital's legal responsibility to ensure the client's communication needs are met.**

- Some deaf and hard of hearing people have indicated that they will only use the health service for really serious health matters as they have found it a stressful experience they would rather avoid if possible.

Use of genetics services

Despite genetic deafness being one of the most common genetic conditions, very few deaf or hard of hearing adults are referred or seek a referral for genetic counselling. It seems that one of the main assumptions about this is that deaf adults are just not interested in using services. Research by the author has shown that this is just not the case and that when given accurate information about what genetic counselling is and what can be offered, many deaf and hard of hearing adults are interested in using the service. It is possible that given the problems deaf people face in using health services generally, they perceive they

[1] See end of this chapter for details.

will also have a negative experience if they access genetics services too.

> Genetics professionals need to be aware that there is a general dissatisfaction with regard to poor communication with health professionals in general. This appears to be influencing attitudes towards genetics services and the propensity to use these services by deaf and hard of hearing clients.

Knowledge and fears of genetic counselling

It is not unusual for both deaf and hearing people to have limited knowledge of what genetic counselling is and what services are available within Clinical Genetics departments. The words 'genetics' and 'counselling' tied together cause confusion and are often misleading. People may assume that psychotherapy is on offer or that the sole aim of the service is to help people 'cope' with something genetic. Genetic counselling offers information about any inherited condition; such conditions might be evident through different generations of a family, e.g. inherited breast cancer or myotonic dystrophy.

Research by the author has shown that many deaf people are either unaware of what genetic counselling is or have misunderstandings – believing that what is offered routinely and indeed is encouraged is prenatal testing for inherited deafness with selective termination of pregnancy for deaf babies. This is certainly not the case in reality. We have also shown that many deaf people are fearful and even distrustful of genetics services and this is likely to be grounded in the historical perspectives of deafness and eugenics (see later) (Middleton, Hewison et al. 1998). Conversely some deaf and hard of hearing people are extremely positive about genetics services, seeing them as offering information and support for deaf families either wanting, or preferring not, to pass on deafness to their children. The message being delivered here is that there are a multitude of perspectives towards genetics services and it should not be assumed that all people referred will be positive about this.

> Health professionals need to be aware that deaf and hard of hearing people may have different attitudes towards genetics services. Some may feel positive, some neutral and some negative.
>
> As with people in the general population, many deaf and hard of hearing people do not know what genetic counselling is. Thus expectations of what can be offered should be established at the beginning of a consultation.

Any written material for deaf and hard of hearing people about genetic counselling and what to expect from the genetic counselling service could very usefully include an acknowledgement of the fears about the service. Personal experience has shown that the fears are very common and they may hinder the counselling process unless the genetic counsellor brings them out into the open and addresses them. The reason this is important is because inaccurate assumptions may linger and also influence the client's decision-making about certain aspects of their care. For example, a deaf client may turn down the offer of a prenatal genetic test for cystic fibrosis because they wrongly assume that the clinicians will also test for deafness at the same time.

> Health professionals need to be aware that some deaf people have misunderstandings about what genetic counselling is and assume that one of the key aims is to offer prenatal testing for inherited deafness with termination of pregnancy if the fetus is found to be deaf. It can be helpful to reassure deaf clients that this is not a key aim of genetic counselling.

Case study: misunderstandings about genetic counselling

Mandy has a moderate hearing loss and uses speech to communicate. She lives with her husband in the USA. Her newborn son, Bradley, has just been diagnosed as profoundly deaf through the Newborn Hearing Screening Programme. The paediatric audiology team suggest to Mandy that they could refer her and the family to the local regional genetics service for genetic

(*Continued*)

counselling. Mandy is surprised and visibly shocked by this as she says she doesn't need any 'counselling'. She also says that she heard through a TV programme on genetics that it was possible to have a test in pregnancy for deafness and abortion if the baby is found to be deaf. She doesn't want this in a future pregnancy and wrongly assumes that a genetic counsellor would encourage her to have this.

The paediatric audiologist reassures Mandy that the aim of genetic counselling is to offer information and support and that the genetics professionals would not force her to have any testing. The paediatric audiologist asks Mandy whether there are any medical conditions in the family that she is concerned about and she mentions that her cousin has Duchenne muscular dystrophy. The paediatric audiologist tells Mandy that genetic counselling can offer information about this too and can tell her whether she has a chance of having a child with Duchenne muscular dystrophy. Mandy is very keen to know more and asks for a referral to be made.

Current leaflets and DVDs focus on clinical aspects of genetic counselling without addressing the fears, suspicions or misconceptions some deaf people have. Additional literature is needed to complement current documents.

The inadvertently patronising health professional

'Health care providers who harbour conscious or unconscious biases against deaf individuals lack proper training to work effectively with them, do not understand their client's perspective and cannot provide good healthcare.' (Harmer 1999, p98)

With the above in mind, it is therefore very helpful for health professionals to move away from the mindset that a deaf person is disabled, handicapped or deficient in some way. If the health professional sees the person who is deaf as defective, it would naturally elevate the hearing health professional to a superior position as being 'non-defective'. This elevation creates a power differential that can be damaging for both sides. The client may automatically assume the position of 'helpless victim' and the doctor an attitude of 'poor you, how can I make you better?' This power dynamic can become exaggerated and lead to the client who is deaf feeling misunderstood and increasingly helpless and the hearing health professional taking on a more paternalistic and authoritative role. If taken to the extreme this could lead to a victim-and-bully dynamic.

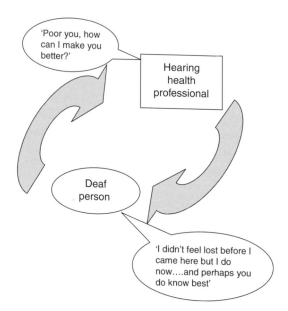

Case study: viewing deafness holistically

Axel is a newly qualified doctor working for 6 months in an Ear, Nose and Throat (ENT) clinic in Denmark. His grandmother became deaf in her 50s and so he is familiar with how disabling a condition this is for her.

Soren is in his 50s and has been losing his hearing since his teenage years. He has a condition called otosclerosis which is caused by hardening of the bones in the middle ear. This can sometimes be successfully treated by surgery. Soren has never really been bothered by his hearing loss. He has a lively sense of humour, a positive attitude and an affable manner. He met and married a profoundly deaf woman in his 20s before he realised and had been diagnosed with otosclerosis himself. The two of them use a mixture of speech, lip-reading and sign language to communicate. They both work for the local council and have quite senior and respected positions. Soren's wife works in services for deaf people and Soren works in Sports and Leisure.

Soren's family doctor suggested he might wish to have a discussion about surgery for his otosclerosis and so he has gone to the ENT clinic to have a chat, but he is not overly keen on having an operation.

Axel meets Soren in clinic to discuss the pros and cons of surgery. Axel knows how successful the surgery can be and feels sure that Soren would have a better quality of life if Soren proceeded with this. He imagines that Soren must struggle to communicate day to day and feels that there is a tangible solution to restore his hearing. Axel assumes that deafness is a problem and being hearing would be preferable.

Soren has never been particularly bothered by his hearing loss, he has always managed to get around it and feels that although it might be irritating for other people, it is part of his identity and he is not sure that he needs to change this. He feels that he can communicate quite effectively with his wife, friends, family and colleagues and this has not held him back in any way. When he hears

(*Continued*)

from Axel what the surgery might involve, he makes his mind up definitely that he doesn't want to proceed.

Axel cannot understand why Soren would turn down the opportunity to restore some level of hearing. He feels sorry for Soren and thinks he is rather misguided. Soren feels annoyed that he cannot just be accepted for who he is and Axel's pity really irritates him.

What could be done differently?

Axel holds a strong unconscious view that deafness is a disability; this is based on his limited experience of his grandmother's deafness. This could be preventing him from seeing Soren as a whole person with a rich and fulfilling life. Axel has a medical perspective of deafness and is not familiar with applying his communication skills to elicit his client's perspective. If Axel was able to reflect on his preconceived ideas about deafness, he may be able to view Soren more holistically.

Qualitative research gathering the views of deaf, sign language users and hard of hearing speech users has shown that deaf and hard of hearing people feel that 'most physicians, largely unconsciously, hold fundamental assumptions about deafness, that, from the outset, undermine client–physician relationships. In particular, physicians do not fully appreciate the totality of patients' lives' (Iezzoni, O'Day et al. 2004, p. 357).

> 'Many physicians hold paternalistic, ethnocentric attitudes towards their patients. Doctors also tend to view disabilities as deviations from the mainstream norm that should be corrected if possible. These beliefs and preconceptions affect both provider and client expectations, interactions, and decisions. Additional problems occur when the physician fails to recognize or appreciate the different frames of reference used by hearing and Deaf individuals when viewing many situations, including health care delivery. Deaf individuals may not perceive hearing loss as a disability and may have different goals and priorities in their health care treatment and their hearing health care provider.' (Harmer 1999, p. 90)

The focus of the following sections moves from the health professional and back to the deaf client. Here we summarise some of the communication methods of relevance to deaf people.

Modes of communication

There are various discrete modes of communication that deaf and hard of hearing people use. The most common of these include: speech, National Signed Language (e.g.

British Sign Language – BSL, Irish Sign Language – ISL), Signed Supported Spoken Language (SSSL), which literally translates spoken language word for word into sign language, while maintaining the same word order as in the spoken language (e.g. Signed Supported English), lip/speech-reading, written notes and speech with finger-spelt cues.

Within a healthcare setting it is particularly important to recognise that fluency in language is not automatically necessary for fluency in communication. This means that body language, facial expression, gesturing and the giving and receiving of non-verbal cues may offer all sorts of information about what a person is feeling more so than language on its own.

Spoken language

The vast majority of people with a hearing loss have mild-moderate hearing loss. Such people will usually use spoken language as their main form of communication. Deafened people also use speech to communicate; this latter group may gain little use from hearing aids and so rely heavily on good communication skills from the person they are talking with. For both these groups of people there is usually a preference for having a healthcare consultation in speech together with a good level of deaf awareness on the part of the health professional (Middleton, Turner et al. 2009) (see later sections for details).

National Sign Language

Although it is socially acceptable for anyone to use sign language these days, it has not always been the case. In relatively recent times it was considered detrimental to the development of speech if sign language was used in education, many schools for deaf children were closed and a more oralist approach was adopted (Ladd 1988). This means that there are profoundly deaf adults who may have benefited enormously from sign language if they had been given access to it. Since they were not they remain on the edges of Hearing society, unable to fully communicate through speech and hearing because of the profound level of their deafness, but also on the edges of the Deaf World because they cannot use sign language.

> National Sign Languages (NSL) and spoken language are not verbatim equivalents. NSLs have their own sentence construction, grammar and word groupings (Fischer and Hulst 2003).

For example, BSL and others, including ASL (American Sign Language), use specific positioning in front of the person signing to construct meaning, and a particular spatial position in conjunction with a sign will denote a specific pronoun (Ralston and Israel 1995). It would be unusual for a person using an NSL to use their voice while they are signing, but they may still mouth some words derived from spoken language at the same time. Therefore, it would be atypical to deliver a spoken commentary while signing in an NSL. This is not the case, however, with Signed Supported Spoken Language (SSSL); because the signing is based on spoken language to start with, it is much easier to sign and speak concurrently.

> National Sign Languages have their own dialects and local variations. For example, the BSLs used in Lincolnshire and Cornwall can be dissimilar at times, in the same way that regional spoken dialects can vary. Also, worldwide, sign languages vary from country to country, as each language has developed independently in the same way that spoken languages have.

When sign language is used, researchers report that different neural patterns are fired within the brain from those used by people speaking (Campbell, MacSweeney et al. 2008). Consequently there could also be different ways of processing memory and learning (Marschark 2003). This means that a deaf sign language user may have no differences in intelligence or educational ability from a speech user, but the way they receive, process and remember information might be different.

Sign Supported Spoken Language (SSSL)

Hearing parents and teachers of deaf children frequently use signs taken from an NSL together with their speech when conversing with deaf children, as National Sign Languages are hard to learn. This is particularly the case if the child with deafness lives amongst a hearing family and sign language is not the main form of communication. This method allows deaf and hard of hearing children to learn to lip-read and also receive signed cues concurrently. SSSL (or Signed Supported English in the UK) tends to bridge a gap between the Hearing and Deaf Worlds and is mainly used by deaf and hard of hearing people who have come to signing later on in life or who mix most of the time in the Hearing World. People who would be considered part of the Deaf culture would usually use an NSL rather than SSSL.

Case study: becoming an SSE user

Marion was born hearing, but after getting meningitis at the age of 7 she lost some of her hearing. She went to a mainstream hearing school in Scotland, but never really felt as if she fitted in as she missed out on many of the conversations that her hearing friends had. Because of this she had hardly any friends at all and she felt really isolated.

At secondary school Marion met another child who had also had a similar experience and they became friends. This other child found a night-school class where it was possible to learn sign language. The class was run by a hearing teacher for deaf children and she taught them Sign Supported English (SSE). As spoken English was already a language they used and they were

(*Continued*)

quite good at lip-reading, the signs were easy to pick up as the teacher mouthed the English word at the same time as teaching the sign.

Within a year both Marion and her friend were fluent in SSE; this opened up a whole new level of communication and they realised that they could now begin to access the Deaf World. Although not fluent in BSL they had enough skills from the SSE to follow BSL conversations. This new language gave them the confidence to seek out others who used SSE and they joined a social club of local hard of hearing people.

Difficulties with speech

Spoken language is sometimes difficult for people with a congenital, profound level of deafness. This is because it is hard for the brain to process the use of sound if the ear has never been able to receive it. Lip-reading and speech-reading for a person who has never heard sound is therefore very difficult (Barnett 2002a). This may be addressed, to a degree, with specific training via education and speech therapy (Kaplan, Gladstone et al. 1993 in Ralston and Israel 1995).

Children from Deaf families who have been raised using sign language as their main form of communication may not experience the concepts of speech until they start school.

This may also be true for hearing children of deaf parents who have had little exposure to spoken language prior to starting school. Research has shown that it is possible for a hearing child to develop normal speech and language from within a Deaf family if they have interaction with hearing speakers approximately 5–10 hours per week (Schiff-Myers 1988 in Israel and Arnos 1995).

This means that, within a healthcare setting, very little communication through the spoken word may be possible. Therefore, it is vital that effective interpretation and/or communication support is available. Not only should this be for the actual clinic consultation, but also during pre-clinic contact with the reception and appointment staff.

Some people who have profound deafness may have received a high level of speech therapy as a child and thus may give the impression of good spoken skills. However, this has the potential to be misleading, as despite having the ability to use clear speech with excellent voice control, they may find it difficult to follow and receive speech in the same effortless manner. Consequently, it should not be assumed that the person who is deaf understands everything that is being said to them and it is the health professional's responsibility to make sure that a two-way conversation is facilitated. Frequently asking the client to indicate whether they are following what is being said is important.

Case study: mismatch in receiving language

Yves lives in France with his wife Constance. He attends a pregnancy booking appointment with his wife. When he speaks to the midwife his voice sounds monotone and she can tell immediately that he is deaf. He talks very articulately at the beginning about how delighted he is that Constance is pregnant and how much he is looking forward to the birth of their new baby.

The midwife begins to talk to Yves and Constance (who is hearing) about the pregnancy and possible screening tests. She directs her conversation mainly to Constance and she gets the impression that Yves must be following what she is saying as he is nodding as she is talking. Yves quietens down and when she asks at the end whether there are any questions, Yves does not answer. The midwife asks again whether there are any questions and Yves says that he didn't follow any of the conversation and asks what she was talking about. The midwife had misunderstood the cues she was getting from Yves and had assumed that just because she could easily understand his speech that he could understand hers.

Comments

The midwife needed to adapt her communication style with Yves. This could have involved paying particular attention to using clear lip-patterns, facing him all the time so that she could be clearly seen, stating at the beginning what she was going to talk about and highlighting when she was going to change topic, rephrasing key messages and checking understanding throughout. She also should have checked at the beginning as to whether he was happy to just lip-read or whether he needed a lip-speaker or other sort of interpreter present.

It is also not uncommon for some deaf and hard of hearing people to give cues that are interpreted by a hearing person as meaning that they understand; for example, nodding. However, this may be misleading and a hearing person may wrongly assume there is more understanding than is actually the case.

Lip-reading

Lip-reading is difficult to do clearly as identical lip-patterns are often used with words which incorporate different sounds from the throat; these may be invisible to the viewer.

Lip-readers develop the ability to utilise many additional factors, such as tongue and jaw movements, gesturing and facial expressions to help with their understanding; collectively this is also known as speech-reading (Kaplan, Bally et al. 1987 in Ralston and Israel 1995).

Many words and sounds look exactly the same on the lips but may have completely different meanings. In fact less than 30% of English sounds can be clearly lip-read (Harmer 1999). For example, it is

(*Continued*)

virtually impossible to lip-read a difference between 'fifteen' and 'fifty' (Harmer 1999). 'Where there's life there's hope' and 'where's the lavender soap' is another example of messages that are incredibly difficult to discern without the help of the voice.

The importance of giving clear lip-patterns is therefore obvious when communicating with lip-readers. This also includes not obstructing the face, e.g. by covering the mouth with fingers or hair, and not chewing food. Eye contact is also important and it is imperative not to turn away the face to look at a set of hospital records or a computer screen.

Case study: communicating with a hearing aid user

Elaine is Canadian. She started to lose her hearing in her 40s. She finally admitted she couldn't hear well when she turned 50 and asked her GP for a referral to have her hearing checked. She had a moderate, progressive hearing loss diagnosed at the local Audiology department. Elaine had to attend numerous hospital appointments to have a hearing aid fitted and checked and for her case to be reviewed. Once the most appropriate aid was found and was adjusted so that it worked well, Elaine found that she could hear again and was overjoyed that her 'disability' was resolved.

In one of the appointments at the hospital, Elaine arrived by car and couldn't find a parking space, and so she approached a member of the security staff to find out where she should go. The security advisor saw Elaine's hearing aid and assumed she must be deaf or hard of hearing and so spoke to her very slowly, exaggerating his lip-patterns and raising his voice. He had seen his mother speak this way to elderly relatives and so assumed that this was appropriate for Elaine.

Elaine winced as her hearing aid amplified this sound; she could hear him perfectly without his needing to speak louder. In addition to this the exaggerated lip-patterns were most unhelpful as they distorted his speech. Elaine said to the security advisor that she could hear him fine without his needing to change anything in the way he spoke, but she did say it was helpful if he faced her so that she could see what he was saying. They then continued to have a pleasant conversation about the difficulties of parking at the hospital.

Comment

A hearing aid user relies on a whole mixture of skills when listening to someone using speech. Not only are they utilising the amplified sound via the hearing aid, but they are also using visual information, gained through non-verbal cues, for example via the expressions on the speaker's face as well as their lip movements. Exaggerated lip-patterns and an increase

(*Continued*)

in volume may not only interfere with the way the hearing aid amplifies speech but may also distort the lip-patterns, so affecting how these are read. There are many hearing aid users who can cope fine with just their hearing aid alone, but it is still helpful to offer additional communication support through paying extra attention to helping with lip-reading.

One factor that significantly helps lip-reading is being able to predict what the conversation will be (Harmer 1999). For example, if waiting in a queue at a fast-food restaurant it is predictable that the first question from the staff will be 'what can I get you today?'

It is therefore helpful in a conversation with a lip-reader to offer signposting to the conversation. For example, 'I'm going to ask you about your diagnosis first then we can discuss your treatment options'.

Reading/writing skills

As signed languages are not a literal translation of written and spoken language, deaf sign language users may find it difficult reading written text as this is in their second language and they will have to translate it. These difficulties are in no way due to intellectual incompetence but more probably due to difficulties in receiving the most appropriate education to overcome such issues. This is an incredibly important point for clinicians to recognise, particularly if they are looking to see whether there is a syndromal cause for the deafness in the client they are seeing – it is very relevant to know whether the person who is deaf has learning difficulties. They may inadvertently assume they do, on sight of some written material in the deaf person's writing, when in fact the person who is deaf is just conversing in their second language.

Research from Europe and the USA indicates that deaf children of deaf parents achieve more educationally than deaf children of hearing parents (Stephens 2005). This has been confirmed by a recent large-scale study in the UK (Fortnum, Barton et al. 2006). The reasoning behind this finding is that deaf parents offer positive role models to deaf children and also have prior knowledge of how to solve communication problems. They also know more about deaf education than most hearing parents do because they have personal experience of it themselves. All these factors appear to influence better academic achievement for deaf children.

Written materials provided for deaf clients should be considered carefully for ease of translation into sign language. Where it is not possible to use anything other than something written down, this needs to be structured in plain English and thought needs to be given to the sentence construction (keep sentences short without meandering) and language use (no jargon).

There are companies that will translate written material into plain English specifically for sign language users for a fee (see list of websites at the end of the book). Where possible, written materials should also be provided on DVD in sign language. Again there are companies that will create such DVDs within a 24-hour turnaround time.

> The genetic counselling team at St Mary's Hospital in Manchester, UK, set up a specific clinical service for deaf clients and their families. They appreciated that the department's existing written leaflets giving details about the clinic and what to expect from the service were not immediately accessible to their deaf clients who used sign language as their first language. They therefore employed a team of Deaf interpreters to translate the written text into BSL. These translations were videotaped and back-translated by an expert in sign language to check for accuracy and understanding. A DVD and video were then created to hand out to potential clients delivering the information in BSL together with a voice-over in spoken language and subtitles (Belk and Middleton 2004, Belk 2006). This is a very useful tool for providing equal access to services and also complies with the UK Disability Discrimination Act (1995).

Not only should client information be provided in plain English or in an NSL on DVD, but so too should consent forms and questionnaires that are used to collect client information, for example the Cancer Family History form often used within genetic counselling.

Using written notes in a consultation can be incredibly helpful for people who use speech as their main language. However, for those who use sign language, written notes in a consultation may be more of a hindrance as the person may struggle to read and process them.

A busy health professional is also likely to write in a briefer manner in a written note, given the time it takes to write one, than they would be if they were explaining in speech (Harmer 1999). This means that a deaf person, particularly a sign language user, is receiving their medical information not only in a language they do not routinely use, but also in a shorter form than their hearing counterpart would receive. It is not difficult to see that this means a substandard service is being provided.

If a client uses sign language as their first language there is no excuse whatsoever for not booking a sign language interpreter for the healthcare consultation.

Meador and Zazove give an example of what happened in a surgical consultation when no interpreter was booked and the Deaf sign language user had to try and communicate by translating the doctor's handwritten notes:

(*Continued*)

'The physician wrote, "You may need surgery". The client understood this to mean, "You need surgery in May". In ASL, the English sentence, "You may need surgery" would be signed, "You maybe need surgery". In ASL, the English sentence, "You need surgery in May" could be interpreted as "You (in) May need surgery." '
(Meador and Zazove 2005, p. 219)

Hearing Dogs for Deaf People

Hearing Dogs for Deaf People are working dogs that assist their owner by alerting them to specific sounds, e.g. the telephone ringing or a tannoy announcement. In the UK the owner has a right to bring them into any public place, including hospitals and health settings where their owner may need assistance. When working they should not be petted nor given any specific attention. However, offering them a bowl of water is acceptable, just in the same way as one might offer a hearing interpreter a glass of water while they are working!

In the UK, Hearing Dogs for Deaf People wear a burgundy jacket, whereas dogs working for other groups, e.g. for disabled or blind people, wear different-coloured jackets.

Planning a deaf-friendly service

If health professionals are planning on overhauling their current environment so that it better suits their deaf clients then it would be most helpful to do this with input from the client group who are going to use it. In order to do this properly it may be appropriate to bring in an external, deaf awareness or deaf equality consultancy service to look at what is currently available and make recommendations. Those companies that are run by deaf consultants and provide training by deaf people are often the most enlightening. Another related nuance is that deaf sign language users will have slightly different awareness needs from hard of hearing speech users and so consideration should be given to this.

> Recommendations may include a financial investment to provide video-telephones, a minicom,[2] a designated phone that can send and receive text messages and access to the Internet. Internet access could provide access to email, MSN messenger, Sightspeed and Skype[3] as well as online interpreting services.

---

[2] The minicom is a telephone used by deaf and hard of hearing people, using written text as the mode of communication. In the past, it was recommended that organisations interfacing with deaf and hard of hearing members of the public should all have a minicom; however, more recently it has become recognised that many deaf and hard of hearing people prefer to use mobile phone texting or emails. If the hearing staff are not familiar with using a minicom and deaf clients prefer to use other forms of communication then the minicom may be a pointless expenditure.

[3] MSN messenger, Sightspeed and Skype are all examples of software that allow video-conferencing to take place over the Internet. Thus they are ideal ways for sign language users to communicate visually without the need for written language.

Such services could be used for booking appointments instead of using a telephone service. It is important to offer a choice of communication methods, for example, making email and texting available to book clinic appointments. It may also be necessary to fit a visual noticeboard, for example, to indicate when the next appointment is ready, in addition to an induction loop for hearing aid users.

> Together with the practical items that should be installed it would also be important for all front-line administration staff, including the receptionist, who is the first person all clients see when they walk in the front door, as well as the administrator who books the clinic appointments, to receive some deaf awareness training.

Again, this can be organised by an external consultancy or there may even be in-house training if the department is in a large, teaching hospital, which is likely to have a designated disability awareness officer. Deaf awareness training is obviously of the utmost importance also for the clinical staff too. Refresher courses should be available to update skills and make sure that new staff are trained.

Before the healthcare consultation

It is important to appreciate that a deaf person cannot begin to communicate if they cannot see the health professional or the interpreter (Barnett 2002a). This means that if they are waiting in the waiting room they will not hear their name being called out and will not pick up cues that it is their turn unless specific eye contact is given, perhaps by the receptionist or health professional approaching them directly when it is their turn.

Alternatively, visual cues can be used. For example, a number could be assigned to each client as they arrive; this number could then be displayed clearly in the waiting room when it is the client's time to be seen. Alternatively an electronic noticeboard could be used, where the client's name is shown as soon as their consultation is ready. This latter approach can work effectively but may not be completely satisfactory as all clients' names are very publicly declared to all present, which could be seen as breaking a level of confidentiality. Another effective tool could be to give each client a pager on arrival in the clinic which then vibrates when it is their turn to see the health professional.

> A very simple solution to help deaf and hard of hearing clients in the waiting room is to position all the seats so that they face the reception or the visual board so that it is very easy to just look up and see what is going on.

If the client is waiting in a consultation room and the health professional needs to enter, the client may not hear a knock on the door and so it is important for the health professional to gently open the door and establish eye contact before entering (Barnett 2002a). It is also pivotally important that, if a physical examination is necessary, eye contact is established first so that the client is not suddenly surprised (Barnett 2002a).

Medical records should be clearly marked with the communication requirements of the deaf or hard of hearing client. In written medical records this could take the form of a bulleted list on the front cover, written in large type, which says, for example:

- Profoundly deaf
- Uses British Sign Language or uses a hearing aid and lip-reading
- Likes to use interpreters from local agency (tel. no . . . . . .)

Alternatively, if the medical records are electronic then it should be possible to put the above list on an auto-alert so that each time any computer entry is made against this client's name, their communication needs are given.

Preferences for communication in a clinical setting

Recent research has shown that Deaf people who use sign language have different preferences for communication in a clinic from those who primarily use speech as their first language (Dye and Kyle 2001, Middleton, Turner et al. 2009). This work shows that very few Deaf sign language users want a consultation in speech; most prefer to either use an interpreter or to have a consultation directly with a signing health professional. Hard of hearing speech users may be content to have consultations in speech but only if there is a good level of deaf awareness on the part of the health professional. Very few speech users indicate they can cope with a consultation in speech alone that lacks deaf awareness (Middleton, Turner et al. 2009).

> Health professionals need to be aware that there are a variety of ways that Deaf sign users and hard of hearing speech users prefer to communicate within a clinic setting.

Deaf awareness

There are a large number of publications indicating that health professionals consistently lack deaf awareness skills (Steinberg, Sullivan et al. 1998, Harmer 1999, Munoz-Baell and Ruiz 2000, Ubido, Huntington et al. 2002, Iezzoni, O'Day et al. 2004, Meador and Zazove 2005, Steinberg, Barnett et al. 2006). The Royal National Institute for Deaf People in the UK has indicated that action is needed urgently to address this (RNID 2004b). However, such action does not seem to have been taken. Despite calls for health professionals to receive deaf awareness training (Department of Health 2005) it does not appear that this is happening in reality.

One of the biggest obstacles for health professionals is recognising that a client is deaf or has a hearing loss. This is particularly relevant for people who don't wear a hearing aid or who have not yet acknowledged that they are losing their hearing. The health professional therefore needs to pay specific attention to assessing whether their client understands the communication.

Steven Barnett from the University of Rochester has written an excellent paper on 'Communication with Deaf and Hard of Hearing People: A Guide for Medical Education' published in *Academic Medicine* in 2002. He summarises the deaf awareness skills needed when communicating with different groups with deafness and this is quoted below (some of the language has been adapted for a UK audience).

Deaf awareness for deaf sign language users

Greeting

Welcome the client with a sign language greeting (or ask the client to teach you one).

Ask the client how best to communicate with him or her.

Environment

Room is well lit, and the light is not shining in the client's eyes.

People are positioned so that the client who is deaf can see the doctor and the interpreter.

Expressive communication

Work with a qualified interpreter.

Speak to the client, not the interpreter.

Topic changes are stated explicitly.

Note-writing and written materials may have limited usefulness.

Ask the client periodically about the quality of the communication.

Ask the client for periodic summaries to check accuracy of communication.

Receptive communication

Look at the client while listening to the interpreter.

When uncertain, ask the client (not the interpreter) for clarification.

Summarise the client's story to check accuracy.

(Barnett 2002a, p. 696)

Deaf awareness for hard of hearing speech users

Greeting

Ask the client how best to communicate with him or her.

Environment

Background noise is minimised.

[Health professional's] face is well lit.

Expressive communication

Eye contact is established before speaking.

View of mouth is not obscured (by hands, pens, charts etc.).

Adjust voice pitch if this helps.

Topic changes are stated explicitly.

(Continued)

Repeat information that is not understood. Rephrase if it is still not understood.

Use assistive listening devices (e.g. hearing aids, note-takers) if they help.

Note-writing may be helpful.

Ask the client periodically about the quality of the communication.

Ask the client for periodic summaries to check accuracy of communication.

Receptive communication

When uncertain, ask the client to repeat or clarify.

Repeat the client's statement to confirm comprehension.

If still unclear, note-writing may help.

Summarise the client's story to check accuracy.

(Barnett 2002a, pp. 695–6)

Case study: the importance of seeing the health professional's face

Helene was in the delivery suite of her local hospital about to give birth to her first child. The obstetrician felt the labour was not progressing as well as it might and that an emergency caesarean was necessary.

Helene was wheeled on her bed into an operating theatre and the medical staff began to put their gowns on. The obstetrician and anaesthetist both put their masks on and neither realised that Helene had a mild-moderate level of hearing loss and prior to this had been lip-reading them.

They were now in an urgent situation, which was made even more frightening for Helene as suddenly she had lost communication with the two key health professionals caring for her.

She was unable to consent to the epidural as she couldn't see the anaesthetist asking her about this and it was only when her husband stepped in and asked the doctor to remove his mask did they realise how significant this was.

Comments

One of the theatre nurses could have taken the initiative and stood in view of Helene, and she could have repeated what the medics were saying with clear lip-patterns. In such an urgent situation, when the medical priority is to deliver the baby and keep the mother safe, there is often no time to make large adjustments to allow for communication access. However, it would not have been too difficult for a member of staff to spend time with Helene, speaking to her face-to-face, to enable her to continue to participate in her care. The level of Helene's hearing loss should also have been noted by health professionals before an urgent situation developed.

In addition to deaf awareness training there is also deaf equality training, which has an emphasis on meeting the requirements of the disability legislation. There are companies that will tailor the training to the specific needs of the client (see websites at the end of the book). For example, GP practice managers and clinic receptionists would be given slightly different information on what needs to be provided in order to comply with the Disability Discrimination Act in the UK.

Communication in a clinical setting

In order to comply with disability legislation, health service providers must make all attempts to meet clients' communication needs. This means the provision of various aids for deaf people, such as investing in an induction loop for hearing aid users, allowing clinics to be booked via text or email and having access to online interpreters.

It also means using the preferred sort of interpreter, and not just booking one who uses an NSL. As will be explained below, there is a large difference between interpreters and communication support staff who use an NSL, SSSL, lip-speakers, note-takers and speech-to-text reporters and it is pivotal to pick the right one.

The client should be consulted about their preferences for type of interpreter but also, where possible, they should be informed of the name of the interpreter. Interpreters are often well known within the Deaf community (as they may also be hearing children of deaf parents) and sometimes, particularly for a healthcare consultation, the client who is deaf may prefer to use someone they already know. Alternatively, they may have strong preferences to only use someone who is unknown to them. Deaf clients also may prefer to book and bring their own interpreter. They may also prefer to have a specific gender of interpreter, for example, if the consultation is in a gynaecology clinic.

> The healthcare service should always cover the cost of the interpreter's fees and travel and sometimes this may also include a booking fee if an agency is used.

Hearing children from deaf families are often used as informal interpreters for their parents. Whilst this may be the parent's choice out of desperation or lack of knowledge of interpreter provision, health professionals should resist this. The mental well-being of any child under the age of 16 should be paramount as they need to develop their own identity and establish a balance between the Deaf and Hearing Worlds (Myers and Marcus 1993 in Israel 1995). It is also possible that using a child as the interpreter will mean that biased information is delivered to the parent (Barnett 2002a), as the child may feel they need to protect the parent or shield them from some information. The

Deaf parent may also not wish to disclose sensitive information in front of their child.

> Health professionals need to ask clients which communication methods they prefer to use in a clinic consultation; they also have a legal obligation to make attempts to meet these.

Types of interpreter and communication support

There are several different ways of interpreting information that are used to support communication for deaf and hard of hearing clients. For example, an interpreter might interpret information between an NSL or an SSSL and spoken language. Alternatively a 'communication support professional', such as a lip-speaker, can convert from spoken language into clearer spoken language and a speech-to-text reporter (STTR) converts speech into written text.

Finally, deaf relay interpreters may be used who convert sign language given by a hearing interpreter and turn this into a more personal sign language that is tailor-made for the client. This is particularly useful for deaf clients who perhaps have very little medical knowledge or language or who have visual problems and are unable to follow a hearing interpreter they do not know or one who is not used to working with visual disability. The way this works is that the clinician speaks, the hearing interpreter interprets this into an NSL and the deaf interpreter translates the NSL into a more accessible NSL. The reason a deaf relay interpreter is useful is because they may have particular knowledge or understanding of an individual deaf client and the way they specifically receive signs.

Working with interpreters

As interpreters often work in many different settings, for example, in social services, the legal system or in signing performances at the theatre, it is vitally important to clarify that they are comfortable working in a medical situation.

> If the health professional has not worked with an interpreter before or has not worked with a specific interpreter who has been booked for a consultation, it is pivotal to arrange a pre-clinic contact either in person or over the phone to discuss what to expect of the consultation.

A rehearsal of the language to be used is of paramount importance so that the interpreter can check their own understanding and practise the phraseology they plan to use. It is not necessary for the health professional to divulge copious amounts of private medical information about the client who is deaf ahead of the consultation. However, particularly if startling or unexpected news is to be conveyed, it can be helpful to forewarn the interpreter of this so that they can be prepared to deliver this information exactly as the health professional intends.

> When working with interpreters, it is important for the health professional not to presume that all of their words and gestures will be translated word for word or even concept for concept with the same tone and inflection of speech.

There are likely to be some differences, and it is important to keep an eye on the interpreter so that it is possible to see whether they are keeping up and whether it would be useful to slow down. It is worth pausing between changes in topic so that there is time for the interpreter to catch up and also so they can indicate such a change to the client. The hearing health professional needs to be aware of working *with* the interpreter so that together they can get across the messages that the clinician intends.

> It is not unusual for a deaf client to sometimes look to the interpreter for support or comfort, almost as if the interpreter is their ally and advocate. This is not the interpreter's role and in the healthcare setting it is the health professional who needs to be supporting the client if this is needed.

The process of interpretation of NSL into speech involves a complex process of reading the signs used, facial expressions (which offer grammatical information) as well as spatial positioning of the hands and body. The interpreter may sometimes have to 'fill in the gaps' of what is being signed to make sense of the message in spoken language.

> Inexperienced interpreters can sometimes succumb to the subconscious pressure from a vulnerable client to support them; this may mean that they 'fill in the gaps' in the interpreting process more than usual, trying very hard to make sense of what a deaf client is signing. However, if that deaf client has mental health or psychiatric issues then it is vitally important that no gaps are filled in and that the interpretation is as true to what the deaf client is expressing as possible.

For this reason it is therefore very important for health professionals to discuss this issue before a consultation and also have a de-briefing session after the client has left to clarify whether the interpreter feels that the client is confused or talking in riddles.

The RNID and British Deaf Association (BDA) provide several factsheets on working with interpreters (see www. rnid.org.uk and www.bda.org.uk). The following sections are based on this information and full credit is given to these organisations for this.

Most UK hospitals have access to registered interpreters through an agency they have a contract with. However, it may be preferable to get to know and use the local freelance interpreters, who usually charge less than agencies. Agencies may also send a different interpreter for each consultation, whereas getting to know a local freelancer may mean that there is an opportunity to build a stronger rapport and thus a greater knowledge base of what exactly is required. A consultation that is expected to last more than 30 minutes may require two interpreters due to the demanding nature of the work. The normal pattern is that interpreters require a break approximately every 30 minutes.

In addition to discussing the content of the consultation with the interpreter prior to the client arriving, it is also expected that there would be a discussion about the seating arrangements within the room. This would involve consideration of the acoustics, position of the light so as to ensure they and the health professional are not in shadow, ensuring there is enough space for hand movements and making sure that the health professional and interpreter can be seen at the same time.

The British Deaf Association recommend that health professionals allow at least 8 weeks to book an interpreter; if there is less time than this then it is likely that interpreters will already be booked. As well as requiring an overview of the general themes to be discussed prior to the pre-clinic contact, interpreters will also need to know the number of people who are deaf and the number of people who will be attending the consultation. The BDA also suggest the following protocol for using an interpreter (British Deaf Association 2005).

- Talk directly to the Deaf person. Correct: 'Did you have trouble finding us today?' Incorrect: 'Please ask if s/he had trouble finding us today.'
- The spoken side of the interpretation is called the 'voice-over' and will always be in first person, e.g.: 'I had no trouble finding you; your directions were very clear.' The Deaf person is 'speaking' with the interpreter's voice.
- Look at the Deaf person and not the interpreter. Maintaining good eye contact will reinforce the feeling of direct communication.
- The interpreter will not take part in the discussion, and is impartial. During the communication, do not ask an interpreter for their opinion or advice.
- The interpreter relays what they hear, so the Deaf person has full access to all communication. Do not say anything you don't want everyone to know!
- The interpreter will interrupt if they need something to be repeated or clarified. Equally, if you are not sure of something, you can ask the Deaf person to repeat or rephrase it. If you think the interpreter may have misunderstood or missed something, it's fine to ask to go back and find out for sure.

(*Continued*)

- Position the interpreter close to the main speaker if possible, and clearly visible to the Deaf person. The interpreter should be well lit, but not from behind – so do not put them in front of a bright window!
- Don't be put off if the Deaf person doesn't watch you when you are talking, because they'll be watching the interpreter.
- The interpreter can only listen to or watch one person at a time, so – as with any communication – it is important to take turns and not talk over each other.
- Speak clearly at your normal pace. Interpretation is almost simultaneous, but there will be a slight delay as the interpreter picks up the meaning of a phrase. If you usually speak very quickly, you may need to slow down a little (the interpreter can advise you). Allow time for Deaf people to respond or ask questions.
- Afterwards, as part of the feedback process, check with the Deaf person whether interpreting arrangements were satisfactory, and whether they would be happy to use the same interpreter again. If you have suggestions for improvement, tell the interpreter or the agency.

(British Deaf Association 2005)

- Interpreters are highly qualified professionals who spend many years training to achieve acknowledged qualifications, for example via the UK organisation Signature (which used to be the Council for the Advancement of Communication with Deaf People).

- There are some who do not achieve such standards who advertise themselves as available to interpret but they have only completed a BSL Level 2 training (intermediate). A sign language user with this level of training is unsuitable to interpret for a medical consultation and should not use the term 'interpreter'.
- It is very important to book an interpreter who is, for example, registered with the National Registers of Communication Professionals Working with Deaf and Deafblind People (NRCPD; relevant for interpreters from England, Wales and Republic of Ireland). Other countries will have similar registers of interpreters.
- Signature have an online directory of qualified interpreters and communication support professionals for the UK (see www.signature.org.uk), which includes: BSL/English interpreters, lip-speakers, speech-to-text reporters, electronic and manual note-takers and LSPs – Deafblind Manual. This latter communication involves using a 'deafblind manual alphabet' and spelling out words and visual information onto the deafblind person's hand. There are qualifications and a register of professionals from each of these categories. There are likely to be similar organising bodies elsewhere around the world.

When looking through the Register of BSL/English interpreters in the UK, choose someone who is a full member, i.e. not a 'junior' or 'trainee' member. A full member will be fully experienced in working in sensitive situations, as found in healthcare.

Lip-speakers

'Lip-speakers' are 'communication support professionals' who help deafened and hard of hearing people who prefer to use speech to communicate. They do not use their voice but mouth the words being said by the hearing person, using very clear lip-patterns and often with the addition of finger-spelling and use of single finger-spelt letters. Everyday speech uses up to 200 words a minute; this may mean that it is difficult for a person who is lip-reading at this speed to absorb all that is said. The lip-speaker will often use fewer words but with the same meaning. As with other forms of communication support this is very skilled and extensive training is required.

Text-based communication support

The RNID have produced an excellent series of information leaflets on the options for assisting deaf people with communication (see www.rnid.org.uk). The following sections summarise some of these leaflets and credit is given to the RNID for this.

Translating spoken language into written text can take several different forms. An electronic note-taker uses a computer to type up a summary of the spoken conversation; not every word is turned into written text. There is usually a time-delay between the speech and the written notes appearing. It is possible to network another computer to the note-taker's so that the person who is deaf can join in with a text conversation. In the UK, if the note-taker uses RNID SpeedText® then a real-time conversation can occur, as every word can be typed without the need to summarise it.

Speech-to-text reporters (STTR) enter words phonetically into a software program and these are then converted into full written text. This enables the reporter to deliver text in real time without delay although it requires high-speed reading in order to keep up. STTRs use Palantype® or Stenograph® in the UK; these are both trade names for the specialised keyboards and associated software used by the STTR.

There is discussion within the interpreting arena as to whether lip-speakers and others who convert, for example, spoken English into other forms of English are actually 'interpreting' as such. What lip-speakers and note-takers do is re-present English in a different English format, whereas with interpreting, for example, from BSL into spoken English, the interpreter uses his or her skills to create the most accurate interpretation of what is being signed, reading facial expressions and body language in addition to the actual signs being used.

Online interpreters

When face-to-face interpreting is not feasible, perhaps because a previously booked interpreter has cancelled at very short notice or because the hospital appointment is likely to be very short, online interpreting can be very useful. It is by no means a substitute for having a face-to-face contact, but it is certainly very helpful when the alternative is to have no interpreter. All the health professional needs is access to a computer, webcam or even videophone.

For access to interpreters via the web there are companies that provide live online interpreting (see websites at the end of the book for details).

Communication over the telephone

Relay telephone systems (e.g. Text Relay in the UK) use an operator to type speech from a hearing person which is then relayed to the person who is deaf via their minicom or computer. The minicom is a telephone which uses text instead of speech as the form of communication and is still used by some deaf people (particularly those from an older generation). Over the last 20 years there has been a great expansion in the technologies available to support and enable d/Deaf people in their communication; see

Harkins and Bakke (2003) for an overview. This technology should be incorporated into clinical practice and more importantly a choice should be offered.

> It is not unusual for deaf people to have very high levels of technological literacy. This may involve the routine use of the iphone and Blackberry to check emails on the move or use of the Internet and a webcam at home. Text messaging received via a vibrating alert is part of daily life; videophones/video messengers, such as MSN messenger, Skype or Sightspeed (a video-conferencing facility), offer easy methods of contacting deaf clients via a computer.

Voice-to-text software

The use of voice-to-text software in a healthcare setting is becoming increasingly popular; as the technology continues to improve it is likely that it will become much more widely available. Not only can it be used to help the health professional with dictation and writing up post-clinic notes, it can also be used in the actual consultation to help people who have difficulty hearing what is being said. All that needs to be done is to position the computer screen so that it can easily be seen by the client, minimising glare from a window or overhead light, and change the size of the text so that it is large enough to be clearly read.

Chapter 3

Specialist issues relevant to working with d/Deaf clients

Anna Middleton

Medical or cultural model?

Medical model

- Deafness is viewed through the 'pathological' or 'medical' model as a medical problem within the ear that needs solving.
- Health professionals tend to use the medical approach to deafness, seeing the need for a hearing aid or a cochlear implant, the assumption being that the client who is deaf or hard of hearing wishes to treat this.

Case study: hearing loss seen as a disability

Bernice is in her late 50s. She started losing her hearing as a child and has grown up as a hard of hearing person in the Hearing World. She uses speech to communicate, but doesn't feel that many people

Working with Deaf People – a Handbook for Health Professionals, ed. Anna Middleton. Published by Cambridge University Press. © Cambridge University Press 2010.

(unless they know her well) understand her. She never learnt sign language because when she was a child it was thought that deaf children only developed cognitively if they focussed on speech rather than sign and in those days sign language was not seen as very politically correct. Bernice feels very strongly that her deafness is a disability and she regularly attends her local audiology department to have her hearing aids checked and evaluated. Her hearing aids are her lifeline and without them she feels she would not be able to communicate at all.

Comment

Bernice views her hearing loss from the medical model. She seeks out health professionals who can try and treat the deafness. Despite the fact that sign language is no longer thought to adversely affect cognitive development, there are still people like Bernice who eschew using it at all and would be perturbed if it was used with them.

Case study: having a cochlear implant

Deepak has a profound, sensorineural hearing loss that has been progressively getting worse recently. He first noticed he was losing his hearing in his mid-twenties and now that he is in his fifties it has become really disabling. He no longer gets any use out of his

(*Continued*)

hearing aids and he is beginning to feel more and more isolated.

Deepak's ENT surgeon suggests he would be an ideal candidate for a cochlear implant and so after discussion with his family he decides he has nothing to lose and so has the surgery. This is a great success and he begins to learn how to hear again and get used to the presence of sound in his life. He has numerous appointments with the speech therapists and gradually over time his own speech returns to how it used to be before he started to lose his hearing; his brain starts to remember and relearn how to process sound. Deepak is delighted his disability has been treated and he feels he can now function well again in the Hearing World.

Cultural model

- The cultural or linguistic model determines that deafness can be viewed differently; here being deaf is tied up with identity and defined by the use of an NSL.
- With the cultural model of deafness it is not a medical problem but more a way of life.

People who are 'culturally Deaf' (written with an uppercase D) feel that they do not have a disability but that it is society's attitudes that are the disabling factor.

- There is a strong identity that comes with using an NSL and Deaf people will often mix with other Deaf people socially and at work.
- It is thought there are somewhere between 50,000 and 70,000 deaf people who use British Sign Language (BSL) as their first or preferred language in the UK and consequently may view themselves as 'culturally Deaf' (RNID 2008).
- Having a strong family history of deafness where sign language is the first language often contributes to a sense of Deaf identity and membership of the Deaf community.

The 'Deaf culture' is international and there are vibrant Deaf communities, for example, in the UK, the USA, the Netherlands, Sweden, Norway, Germany and Australia.

- The Deaf community is also termed the Sign community in the UK.
- Audiological measurement does not determine membership of the Deaf community (Woll and Ladd 2003). However, many culturally Deaf people have a congenital or early-onset, profound level of deafness and hence use sign language. Conversely there are others with this audiological assessment who prefer to identify more with the Hearing World.
- Ninety per cent of Deaf individuals partner other Deaf individuals (Schein 1989).

- Families with a positive Deaf identity may prefer to have deaf children so that they can continue their culture and language in the next generation.
- Seventy per cent of deaf couples who have only deaf children are believed to be deaf because of changes to the GJB2 gene (Nance, Liu et al. 2000).

> Deaf individuals are often interested to know whether and how they have inherited their deafness and what the chances are of passing this on to children (Arnos, Israel et al. 1992). However, they very rarely access healthcare services such as Clinical Genetics to get this information (personal communication from the East Anglia Clinical Genetics Service, Cambridge, and the All Wales Medical Genetics Service, Cardiff, 2008).

Case study: deafness seen as an identity

Miranda is culturally Deaf, she uses sign language as her preferred language and does not perceive her deafness as a problem. She is an excellent lip-reader and also has clear speech and can communicate well with health professionals.

She goes to see her GP because she has just discovered she is pregnant; she is excited about having a baby and as this is her first she wants to ask her GP about antenatal care and the next steps she needs to take to organise this.

The GP welcomes Miranda into her office and offers her congratulations for the pregnancy. After a time she asks Miranda whether she has a family history of deafness and Miranda says quite proudly that she comes from a family with four generations of deafness.

The GP confides that there is a chance that her baby might be deaf too and asks in a concerned voice whether Miranda has considered this. Miranda says 'of course!' and states that if the baby is deaf this will be fine as it will be the same as the rest of the family and actually she would prefer to have deaf children for this reason.

The GP is visibly shocked and says she is surprised that Miranda would want to pass on her disability to her children. Miranda says that she doesn't feel her deafness is a disability and there really is no problem with being deaf.

The GP looks confused and Miranda feels scolded and misunderstood; she wonders how her GP does not know about the sense of pride that culturally Deaf people have in their history, language and community. Miranda leaves the consultation feeling deflated and disappointed.

Comment

It is not unusual for some Deaf people to prefer to have deaf children. Many families have several generations of deafness and a real sense of pride in

(*Continued*)

this. Research has shown that deaf children with deaf parents do better in terms of educational and academic achievements, employment and psychological functioning, when compared with deaf children from hearing families.

It is well known that some deaf families prefer to have deaf children and celebrate the birth of a new deaf baby into the family (Hoffmeister 1985, Dolnick 1993, Erting 1994, Middleton, Hewison et al. 1998). However, the birth of a deaf baby into a hearing family with no knowledge, experience or expectation of deafness can be devastating. Parents may grieve the loss of a child they had been hoping for and have to embrace a whole new mindset as they come to terms with raising a child who cannot hear.

Case study: shock at a new diagnosis

Jerrick and Aretha are both hearing. They have no family history of deafness and do not personally know any deaf people. They are in their early 20s and are the first of their peers to become pregnant. The baby will be the first grandchild for both sides of the family and is awaited with great anticipation and excitement.

After delivering a beautiful baby girl and while still in hospital, Aretha consents to the baby's hearing being tested. She is soon told that the baby has a severe level of hearing loss and that further tests will be needed. Aretha and Jerrick are absolutely shocked to the core; it had never crossed their mind that their baby might be anything but 'perfect'. They were still getting used to the idea of having a baby, let alone a baby with perceived special needs. They are devastated and grieve for the baby that they had thought they were having. It takes them both a long time to accept that their family will no longer be as they had expected. In time they begin to accept that their beautiful baby is still their precious child and that they need to construct a new future for themselves.

Health professionals need to be aware that some deaf people prefer to have deaf children, others prefer to have hearing children; some want deafness to be eliminated and others are appalled by this idea.

Historical context to deafness, eugenics and genetics

There have been many endeavours over the last few hundred years to use perceived knowledge about the inheritance of deafness to negatively influence the reproduction of deaf people.

Assuming that all deaf couples will have deaf children (an inaccurate assumption) has led eugenicists throughout history to create policy that prevented deaf couples from having children. One of the best-known proponents of this was Alexander Graham Bell (inventor of the telephone and also a leader in the eugenics movement), who wrote a paper in 1883 called 'Memoir Upon the Formation of a Deaf Variety of the Human Race' and presented this to the National Academy of Sciences. Within this work he suggested that all deaf people should only marry hearing people rather than deaf people so that deafness could be reduced in society (Bell 1883). He was actually very supportive of deaf people and felt he was doing society a favour as his own experience of deafness in his wife and mother led him to believe that it was a disability to be avoided at all costs. However, his views now hold a place in history as a very negative influence within the Deaf community and as such often become a talking point when issues relating to eugenics are raised.

> Additional events of great historical significance which threatened the Deaf community were the eugenic policies of the Nazis in the Second World War. Seventeen thousand deaf people were specifically targeted as part of the Nazi programme 'Operation T4', where deaf children and adults were forcibly sterilised and killed so that they could not have deaf children (Biesold 1999 in Schuchman 2004).

Both these events relied on the inaccurate assumption that deaf people have deaf children. In fact, recessive deafness is the most common form of genetic deafness and 90% of deaf children are born to hearing parents. The idea that the human race can be 'improved' by using genetic technology or genetic information to stop particular people having children comes under the umbrella of 'eugenics'. Many deaf people mistakenly think that modern-day genetics services follow the same eugenic principles. Indeed, when deaf people are asked their views about current genetics services the issue of prenatal testing and selective termination for deafness often arises. Participants in the most recent research work by the author have indicated there are large misunderstandings about the aims of current genetic counselling services. The actual ethos of existing services is not to give advice nor encourage specific actions to be taken, for example, having a prenatal test for deafness. Indeed prenatal testing for deafness is very rarely requested in genetics services. Many deaf people feel that genetic testing for deafness 'devalues' deaf people (Middleton, Hewison et al. 1998).

> Health professionals need to be aware of the historical context within which modern-day genetics services sit and that some deaf and hard of hearing people may associate genetic counselling with eugenic practices of the past.

Because of the sensitivity surrounding the medical model of deafness amongst some deaf people, it is very important for all health professionals to have an understanding of this. It is one possible explanation as to why some deaf people rarely attend medical appointments.

Planning a deaf-friendly genetics service

In addition to the general guidance above, it is paramount that appropriate members of the genetics team receive deaf awareness training. At the moment, deaf adults very rarely access genetic counselling services; this is due to a number of access issues that are being identified in current research. Once these access issues are addressed it is likely that deaf adults will come for genetic counselling much more frequently, not just to discuss deafness but also to discuss other conditions that might be running through their family. It is paramount that staff know how to work appropriately with this client group.

Training recommendations for staff working in genetics services

- Genetics professionals need to be aware that deaf people are interested to know why they are deaf and whether this can be passed on to their children.
- Genetics professionals need to be aware that deaf people are interested in having genetic counselling for conditions other than deafness.

- Substantial deaf awareness training is recommended for at least one member of administration staff and one member of clinical staff in each genetics department. This training should be offered by someone who is deaf or, if this is not feasible, should have significant input from someone who is deaf.
- All genetics professionals who *regularly* see deaf and hard of hearing clients (for example, on a monthly basis) should have deaf awareness training
- At least one member of the genetics team *frequently* seeing deaf sign language users (for example, as part of a specialist deafness clinic, perhaps on a monthly or even weekly basis) should undertake NSL training at least to a basic level.
- Genetics professionals who specialise in working with deaf clients and who frequently see deaf sign language users should aim for fluency in their NSL and be able to deliver a consultation in NSL.

Practical issues to think about in relation to any healthcare consultation

Each clinical department should discuss practical issues relating to clinic attendance, e.g. use of text messaging and email to arrange appointments and ensuring familiarity with telephone relay services.

Timing of consultations

Consultations that are facilitated by the use of an interpreter may take slightly longer than consultations without an interpreter because the interpreting process of speech into sign may not be in exact real time. This is particularly the case if the health professional is speaking fast or there are several complicated concepts to relay; it is not unusual for the interpreter to need time to 'catch up' with their translation. This means that the health professional should pause every few minutes or so; this could helpfully happen each time there is a shift in topic.

> Good deaf awareness on the part of the health professional will also mean that the main messages of what they want to say are repeated, rephrased and also checked for understanding. This applies both to consultations that are interpreted and also to those that are not, as working with hard of hearing speech users also requires the same consideration.

A client who uses speech may require the health professional to use a mixture of clear (and possibly slower) speech, together with handwritten notes or, if present, electronic notes (see the previous chapter on note-taking). The hard of hearing speech user will need time to lip-read as well as avert their eyes to the written word and then back again.

Any speech delivered by the health professional is wasted while the client who is deaf or hard of hearing is not looking, so there will need to be several pauses while the client is allowed time to move their eyes to the written text and then look back to the health professional.

Case study: communication with an elderly, hard of hearing client

Ivanna is in her 80s and has been losing her hearing over the previous 20 years. She has a severe hearing loss and does not wear a hearing aid. She attends a physiotherapy appointment 6 weeks after a fracture in her hand has healed. The physiotherapist needs to consider carefully how she communicates with Ivanna since Ivanna cannot hear a normal conversation without additional communication help.

The physio sits directly in front of Ivanna, with the light in front of her so that her face is clearly visible. She also makes sure that she meets with Ivanna in a quiet environment where background noise is minimised and they are not likely to be interrupted. She speaks more slowly than she normally would (but is careful not to sound patronising or laboured) and she also uses a louder voice. The physio has a pen and paper to hand so that she can draw and write on it to help support what she is saying and she also makes sure that she

> (*Continued*)
>
> doesn't turn away her face or obstruct her mouth while she is talking. She asks periodically whether Ivanna is following the conversation and frequently summarises what she has said.

The process of trying to follow a mixed form of communication (e.g. lip-reading and following an interpreter or note-taker) is tiring and so it is also important not to allow these appointments to go on too long.

It would be far better to book two 45-minute sessions than expect a deaf client to sit through 1.5 hours in one go. Conversely if the clinic appointment slot is only for 10 minutes, it is likely that this will need to be doubled for a deaf client, to allow for communication issues to be addressed.

> It is vital for health professionals to have flexibility in their appointment system so that if additional time is required for a consultation involving deaf clients, then this can be utilised.

Use of language

All sensitive health professionals should think carefully about the language they use with all of their clients. This is particularly pertinent when working with deaf clients because there is no single way to view deafness – not everyone perceives it as a disability and to those who do, for some it may be more serious than for others. Therefore, any value-laden terms should be avoided. For example, saying to the new parents of a deaf baby, 'I am so terribly sorry to tell you your baby is deaf', may be really overstepping the mark if the family do not see deafness as the end of the world. Conversely it should not be assumed that a deaf person wouldn't perceive their deafness as an absolute tragedy and thus the reverse is just as inappropriate: 'I'm pleased to tell you that the only problem with your baby is that he is deaf'. It is just safest to be as neutral as possible in the language used: 'Our results show that your baby is deaf' and then immediately adjust further responses to the client based on their reaction to the information.

Health professionals need to be aware that, as deaf people may have different views towards having deaf children, they should not use value-laden language when discussing having children.

Case study: joy at the deafness diagnosis

Bruno and Adelle are both deaf sign language users from Germany. They belong to the local Deaf community and have a strong Deaf identity.

They have just had a baby called Ava and have come to their local hospital to see the paediatric audiologist to have Ava's hearing tested. They are excited to know

(*Continued*)

whether Ava is deaf. Bruno comes from a hearing family and Adelle has several generations of deafness in the family.

The paediatric audiologist arranges an NSL interpreter for the consultation. After the testing is complete she gives Bruno and Adelle the results. She starts the conversation by saying, 'I'm so terribly sorry to have to tell you that Ava is sadly deaf'.

Adelle and Bruno smile at each other; inwardly they are delighted with this news, but they do not like to show this too much in case they are seen as uncaring parents. The paediatric audiologist spends the next 10 minutes talking about options for treatment such as a cochlear implant and fitting for a hearing aid. Adelle and Bruno just nod and take the leaflets she provides.

As they leave the consultation room and are in the corridor outside, alone, they hug each other. They can't wait to tell Adelle's family as they know they will be so excited, although they know that Bruno's hearing parents will be disappointed. As they leave the hospital they throw the written material from the health professional in the bin – they can neither understand it as it is in written language nor want it as they do not see Ava as needing to be treated.

Comments

The paediatric audiologist should have used neutral language to deliver the news about Ava, rather than the value-laden words 'I'm so terribly sorry'. If she had also more awareness about Deaf culture she would have known to ask whether they wanted to know about cochlear implants rather than just assuming this. The written material needed to be adapted so it was relevant and sensitive for deaf and hard of hearing people but also written in a manner that could more easily be understood by sign language users.

For those working in a genetics clinic, words such as 'mutation', 'gene fault' and 'risk of abnormality' are often used. However, there is so much scope for mis-translation of these concepts and also risk of offence that it is particularly important to avoid these at all costs. Alternative words such as 'possibility' could be used instead of 'risk' or 'different' instead of 'abnormal'.

Case study: use of sensitive language

Kalina attends a genetic counselling consultation; she is a deaf sign language user. An NSL interpreter has been booked for the consultation. The interpreter arrives late and also had not had any time to discuss possible ways of interpreting genetics concepts before the actual consultation.

The clinical geneticist (doctor) talks to Kalina about the family history of deafness and says that it is likely that there is a mutation in one of the deafness genes that has caused the members of Kalina's family to be deaf. The interpreter doesn't really understand what

(*Continued*)

'mutation' means but doesn't have time to ask so she interprets this as 'mutant deafness'. Kalina sees this and feels very offended that she is being labelled as having 'mutant deafness'. She does not concentrate on anything else the clinical geneticist says in the rest of the consultation as she feels more and more upset about this.

The clinical geneticist is oblivious as to how her speech is being interpreted and if she had known that the word 'mutation' was causing so much concern she would never have used it. It would have been just as easy for her to use the phrase 'altered gene' as this has the same technical meaning.

Comments

The clinical geneticist should have made time to meet with the interpreter first so that she could explain the genetic terminology she intended on using and check the interpreter's understanding of this. She could have also kept a closer eye on the interaction between interpreter and deaf client so that she could pick up from the non-verbal cues that the client was confused and offended by something. The clinical geneticist should also have been aware of the sensitivity to terms such as 'mutation' and used alternatives.

Health professionals need to be aware of the sensitivity some deaf people have towards genetic language. Avoid words such as 'mutant', 'mutation', 'abnormal', 'normal'; be sensitive to words such as 'risk'.

There must be specific training for interpreters working within genetic counselling settings, to enable them to properly discuss genetics issues with deaf clients.

It is not usual for genetic terms to exist in some languages. For example 'recessive', 'gene', 'chromosome' and 'DNA' cannot be literally translated into Urdu as the translations do not make any sense, e.g. 'recessive' translates to 'out of sight' in Urdu (Shaw and Ahmed 2004, p. 330). In a consultation with a deaf person using BSL the same sign may be used by the interpreter to describe several different concepts, e.g. 'chromosome', 'gene' and 'DNA'. This may happen largely because the interpreter has limited genetic knowledge and presumes that these words in spoken English all have the same meaning. The conclusions drawn by Shaw and Ahmed can be applied here. They suggest that it is most helpful to keep the English word and not attempt to translate it directly, but then offer a description in the native language (Shaw and Ahmed 2004). This means in sign language that the genetic term could be finger-spelt first (e.g. c-h-r-o-m-o-s-o-m-e) and then a shorthand sign given to it that denotes this finger-spelt word. The new sign can then be described by the signer, for example, 'chromosome is a word used to indicate a collection of genes, all packaged up on top of each other'. This means that the interpreter must have a medical understanding of the term 'chromosome' and 'gene' first so that they can describe it in BSL (Middleton, Robson et al. 2007). As suggested earlier, this is one of the reasons why it is paramount to have a conversation with interpreters before the consultation so that these sorts of concepts can be clarified.

It could also be helpful to send pictures and descriptions of common medical terms that are likely to be used in the consultation to both the interpreter and the client; this can be done ahead of the consultation.

Taking a family history

Ninety per cent of deaf children are born to hearing parents (Cohen and Gorlin 1995). Hearing parents of deaf children may struggle to communicate with their children as they are growing up and this can sometimes result in a level of emotional detachment, lack of closeness or even feelings of exclusion.

Given the fact that the hearing child may also miss out on many spoken discussions and incidental conversations about the family, it is not unusual for deaf adults from hearing families to have a lack of awareness about specific medical information about their relatives.

They may be unaware of distant relatives with cancer because it was all too easy to miss the family conversation about this. For a health professional needing to collect family history information from a deaf client, it may be necessary to get permission to call their hearing relatives for more data (Israel and Arnos 1995).

Case study: isolation from family information

Trude first shows signs of hearing loss when she is 10 years old. By the age of 15 she has a diagnosed mild-moderate level of hearing loss; she is told that over time her hearing is likely to worsen.

Trude is very self-conscious of her hearing aids and is very shy. The new diagnosis hits her hard and she withdraws from her family and friends. She spends most of her time on the computer in her bedroom. Trude is from a large family and has four other siblings, all of them younger.

Trude finds it difficult to follow conversations in the home as there is usually a lot of background noise. She also finds that it irritates her siblings each time she asks them to repeat something so she has just given up joining in family conversations. This is also the case when other relatives come to stay.

On joining a new GP practice, the practice nurse asks Trude whether she has a family history of heart disease, high blood pressure and cancer. Trude realises that she has absolutely no idea; she has never

(*Continued*)

heard any family conversations about any of these conditions.

Trude also realises how detached she has become from her family. Her hearing loss has brought a distance between them and she resolves to begin to address this. She thinks about the isolation she feels and wonders how her parents have let this happen.

Asking about a family history of deafness

Given the sensitivities surrounding genetics and eugenics it is not surprising that some deaf people who are aware of this history can be a little sensitive about answering questions from health professionals about their family history of deafness.

Many deaf people still view anything about genetics and the inheritance of deafness with suspicion. If a health professional needs to explore a family history of deafness, for example, so that they can rule out a particular syndrome, then they may need to ask explicit information about who was deaf in the family and how this affected the relative. It is therefore paramount that they explain this is what they are doing and the reasoning for this.

Health professionals need to explain carefully why they might need to ask questions about a family history of deafness (e.g. to explore whether there is a syndrome associated with the deafness) since the motives behind this questioning may be misunderstood.

Health-related knowledge

It is not unusual for deaf people to miss out on general health-related information that is available to hearing peers through overheard conversations with family, incidental chat, TV or radio programmes (Rogel 2008). Therefore, basic knowledge about health issues that one might assume everyone has may be missing (Barnett 2002a). For example, Harmer gives details of several studies offering evidence about the lack of specific health information (Harmer 1999, pp. 82–3). Hearing students may have higher levels of knowledge about medical terminology than deaf students and may also know more about dealing with common medical emergencies (Kleinig and Mohay 1991). Deaf adults indicated in a survey that they did not know what normal body temperature was (Lass, Franklin et al. 1978) and were also unable to correctly identify the meaning of words such as 'anxiety' or 'nausea' (McEwen and Anton-Culver 1988).

Case study: knowledge of medical language

Jason was 3 when he was diagnosed as being profoundly deaf. His mother was also deaf and his father hearing. Jason's parents decided that they wanted a specialist, sign language education for him and so when he reached the aged of 7 they sent him to board at a residential school 400 miles away from their home. Jason came home to his family for school holidays and gradually over the years developed into a strong, independent, confident young man.

His time away from home meant that he missed out on family conversations about health and illness; he didn't know his grandmother had osteoporosis or that his brother had dislocated his shoulder. Due to the fact that he was rarely present at home he missed the incidental conversations that used medical terminology.

If ever there was a health issue at school then the nurse dealt with it and in extreme cases the local hospital was involved. It was only when Jason studied biology at school that he became aware of a whole, new medical language that existed. He was fortunate in that this school offered him the opportunity to participate in this academic subject, but many of his deaf peers whom he met later in his life had not had this opportunity and Jason was surprised that they didn't know even very basic medical terms.

In the same way that deaf people may miss out on general health information about themselves and their family, they may also miss out on how to appropriately use healthcare services.

This is particularly pertinent for those deaf people who very rarely use services. For example, they may go to an Accident and Emergency department for a complaint that could be dealt with by a GP or they may bring an urgent medical query to a consultation in Audiology Services. Health professionals should be prepared to direct deaf people clearly to appropriate services, perhaps by making actual referrals or, if already in a hospital setting, walking around to the appropriate department with them so that they can be registered with a different department.

Differences between healthcare culture and Deaf culture

It is usual for health professionals to have certain expectations of how a client should 'behave' in a consultation. For example, they hope that the client will provide the relevant medical information and history in an efficient manner so that they can make a diagnosis. They will be looking out for specific cues to help them to piece together a picture. It is usual, within Deaf culture, to relay a story, using lots of repetition, facial expression and imitation, which may make it difficult for someone unfamiliar with this mode of communication to 'hear' the medical messages (Harmer 1999). This means that 'differing expectations about normal conversation structure may be a cause of confusion' (Barnett 2002a, p. 697).

Kelly Rogel, a deaf genetic counsellor from the USA, has summarised the above nuances (Rogel 2008). She suggests that the sign language story-telling within a health consultation may offer the main message at the beginning, with the explanations surrounding this afterwards. This contrasts with speech, where a hearing person may relay the story in a more linear fashion and build up to the punchline (with key medical cues) at the end. Meador and Zazove report that 'English [*spoken*] communication works its way up to the main point and then concludes; ASL [*signed*] communication starts with the main point and winds down. Therefore, physicians may believe communications are finished when Deaf clients are still "winding down" the conversation' (Meador and Zazove 2005, p. 218). Rogel cites work by Barnet which suggests that speech users will end a conversation quickly whereas sign language users find this rude and may prefer to continue telling the story (Barnett 2002b).

Rogel concludes that there is much scope for misinterpretation of body language too. For example, within the Hearing World, if a person nods their head when someone is speaking to them it indicates that they are agreeing with what is being said, whereas within Deaf culture head-nodding indicates that the sign language user is following what is being said, rather than actually agreeing with it (Barnett 2002b). In addition to this, people with hearing loss who use their residual hearing in communication will often give the impression of following a conversation (by nodding) when in fact they are struggling to hear and therefore understand what is being said, but feel embarrassed about expressing this.

> Health professionals should consider restructuring the conversation with sign language users so that they allow for the main health issues to be discussed at the beginning, with the general chit-chat to happen at the end.
> Health professionals should not assume that a person who is nodding understands what is being said.

A person using sign language integrates non-verbal body language into their communication; this is inextricably linked to the grammar of sign language. For example, variations in facial expression can be used to discriminate between a pain that is mild and a pain that is intolerable. This is one of the features that make sign language so descriptive. Some hearing speech users, who use words to add texture to their descriptions and who do not typically give much away in their facial expressions, may find this unfamiliar territory. As Barnett writes, 'Different interpretations of nonverbal gestures, such as body posture, facial expression and touch can also lead to misunderstandings' (Barnett 2002a, p. 697).

Case study: mismatches in translation

Tom is a consultant radiologist with a very dry sense of humour and a 'dead-pan' manner about him. He is articulate and witty and uses words very cleverly, giving nothing away in his facial expressions. He is sometimes difficult to read in that his colleagues are often not sure whether he is joking or being serious.

Tom meets Sarah, a deaf client who uses sign language. Sarah has found a breast lump that looks very suspicious on the mammogram and Tom will be performing an ultrasound-guided biopsy of the lump. An interpreter has been booked for their consultation. Tom has not worked with any deaf sign language users before and so is unaware that he needs to adjust his communication style.

Tom enters the consultation room and Sarah is lying on the bed with a gown around her, prepared and ready for the procedure; she has already done a lot of reading up about what to expect so she feels confident about what Tom is going to do. Tom knows she is probably nervous and so to break the ice he says with a very serious face, 'don't worry, we won't remove your whole breast on this occasion'. This might have been an opportunity with a hearing client for a smile as his dead-pan manner could be interpreted as quite funny. However, what Tom says is translated directly by the interpreter and Sarah can see from his facial expression that he looks, and therefore must be, serious.

She is confused; she didn't think there was even a possibility that her whole breast would be removed. As Tom approaches her with the ultrasound equipment she jumps away, suddenly feeling very self-conscious. She puts one hand across her breast and with the other signs, 'you are not going to remove the breast are you?' Tom is surprised: how could Sarah have misunderstood his joke? He apologises and reassures her. Sarah spends the rest of the procedure feeling very anxious and unsure whether she can trust this doctor.

What could be done differently?

Tom needed to adapt his expressive communication with a sign language user. He could have checked with the interpreter before the consultation with regard to how his words would be interpreted and the interpreter would also have had a chance to get to know him a little and consequently could have picked up on his dead-pan manner. This shows the importance of having a briefing session with an interpreter before the consultation. This case also shows that deaf sign language users depend on facial expressions for clues about communication and not the voice or words that are used.

When Deaf NSL users communicate with each other, perhaps in a large grouping of several NSL users, it is not unusual for the group to behave differently from the way a speech-using, hearing group of people might. For example, a person who wants to catch someone else's eye may flap their hand in front of the person's face to get their attention or they may stamp their foot so that vibrations can be felt.

> If, in a clinical consultation, there is a family of sign language users all being seen together, it is socially acceptable for the health professional to use a hand wave in front of someone's face to indicate that they need to slow down or to only sign one at a time so that the interpreter can keep up.

- Eye contact is very important in a conversation with a deaf sign language user. It implies that the signer is being given full attention and the recipient is focussing on them. This is still the case if the signers themselves are looking at the interpreter or elsewhere.
- A hearing person who continually looks away while they are communicating or who shuts their eyes to think may be seen by a sign language user as an oddity or as not paying attention or even as being rude.

> Sometimes the deaf or hard of hearing person will stop the conversation and wait for eye contact to be established before resuming what they are saying. This is because it is possible for the deaf person to forget that hearing people can listen to a conversation without also looking at the person they are conversing with.

An inappropriate focus on deafness

> Research has shown that health professionals may sometimes focus too much on deafness in a consultation, particularly when other issues are the reason for referral.

When Iezzoni et al. interviewed deaf and hard of hearing people about their experiences of the healthcare system, they showed that 'respondents wondered why physicians repeatedly question them about what caused their deafness when hearing is irrelevant to their current health concerns'(Iezzoni, O'Day et al. 2004, p. 358). This same finding was evident in the author's latest research on attitudes towards the use of genetics services. Here it was found that deaf and hard of hearing participants reported that their GP as well as other health professionals often focussed more on their deafness than the pertinent health concerns about which they had come to see the health professional.

Case study: not needing to focus on deafness

Li had a family history of young-onset breast cancer in her mother and maternal aunt. She was referred to the local Breast Unit to find out the significance of the family breast cancers.

Li had been profoundly deaf from birth and so too had most of her family. When the breast care nurse drew up the family tree the first question she asked was: 'Is there anyone else in the family who is deaf?' Li wasn't sure of the relevance of this as she had come to discuss breast cancer, but she answered anyway that her parents, her brother and all of her mother's family were congenitally deaf. The breast care nurse seemed excited by this and said, 'Gosh I've never seen such a large family with deafness before!' She then proceeded to colour in the family tree with symbols to indicate who had deafness.

Li became irritated as she didn't want to discuss deafness, she didn't see this as a medical problem that needed to be noted on a medical chart and she was pretty sure this wasn't relevant to the breast cancer. She asked the breast care nurse if there was a link between breast cancer and deafness and the nurse said no. Li then said that she didn't want to focus any longer on the deafness.

Comment

The health professional here is in danger of losing the client's trust, which may affect how they engage with this particular clinical service in the future. It is important to be guided by the client and to make specific attempts to pick up on how they feel about the discussions being had. This can often be done by looking at non-verbal cues the client is giving which indicate frustration or dissatisfaction.

Health professionals need to be aware that some deaf and hard of hearing people may prefer not to focus on deafness within a consultation, particularly if they have been referred because of a different reason.

Visual aids

Deaf and hard of hearing people, both sign language users and speech users, tend to be visual people. They are used to reading language through observation of lip-patterns, gestures, body language, eye contact and a whole range of visual cues. It therefore makes sense to make use of this skill within a healthcare setting.

This can be done via the use of diagrams, models, animations, drawings and hand signals (for example, one hand to indicate a recessive gene and the other a dominant gene).

Repetition and rehearsal

- Using an NSL requires a different memory process from using speech (Marschark 2003).
- Teachers of deaf children have long known this and it is recognised that this can be addressed using repetition and rehearsal (Gibson 2004). This structure should also be adopted within a healthcare consultation.

Case study: visual communication to describe medical terms

Roberto and his wife Maria attend a genetic counselling consultation. They are both profoundly deaf.

Their genetic counsellor, Alison, has established prior to the session that they require a BSL/English interpreter and has booked a local freelance worker who is a full member of the NRCPD (Alison checked through the Signature website).

Alison has already had a long chat with the interpreter on the phone to discuss the sorts of genetic terminology she will be describing in the consultation and how she plans to structure the session.

They have discussed how the interpreter plans to sign particular concepts, such as 'dominant inheritance' and 'gene alteration'. Alison has also given the interpreter a basic biology lesson on what DNA is as well as 'gene' and 'chromosome' and 'genome'. In addition to this she has sent some written information and drawings in the post to the interpreter. Alison has also provided information about the room they will be using and how the light is positioned, and has already given some thought as to where it might be appropriate to arrange the seating.

In the consultation, Roberto and Maria ask for information about the chances of having deaf children. It is clear to Alison that there is a dominantly inherited, genetic deafness on Roberto's side of the family and an environmental cause to Maria's deafness.

Alison first defines the terms she is going to use, 'genome', 'chromosome', 'gene' and 'DNA', and shows the couple pictures of these using a library metaphor – the 'DNA' represents the words in a book, each individual book represents a 'gene', each shelf of books represents a 'chromosome' and a set of shelves represents a 'genome'. She checks that the couple are following her and asks several times for them to give feedback on what she is saying so that she can check their understanding.

When Alison describes 'dominant inheritance' she draws on a piece of paper, being careful to not talk at the same time so that the couple can watch her draw. When they look up she describes what she has drawn. In order to reinforce the points she is making she also describes 'dominant inheritance' using her two hands to represent two genes, she then moves her hands to indicate one gene being passed on and the other not.

(*Continued*)

Alison asks Roberto and Maria to summarise what their understanding of the genetic terminology is and also asks them to draw out the inheritance pattern too.

At the end of the consultation, Alison gives the couple a DVD containing an NSL version of the department leaflet on 'What is dominant inheritance?' so that they have a sign language record of the information.

Comment

Alison has used four different visual methods to relay information – pre-printed pictures, live drawing, hand signals and a DVD summary. This has all been delivered in sign language, with several opportunities to repeat and rephrase the different concepts. The couple's understanding has also been checked throughout the consultation.

A list of NRCPD-registered interpreters in England, Wales and Northern Ireland can be found at www.signature.org.uk.

Psychological impact of hearing loss

An adult who has grown up hearing and using spoken language may find it incredibly difficult to adapt to the development of a hearing loss. It is common for a whole range of emotions to be attached to this: 'embarrassment, loss of confidence, anger and resentment are among the most common feelings they have to deal with everyday' (Munoz-Baell and Ruiz 2000, p. 41).

> The impact of this can mean that such hard of hearing and deafened people find they shy away from public situations, go out less frequently and withdraw from the events in which they would otherwise be involved. Gradually over time this can lead to isolation, depression and loss of self-esteem.

Case study: negative impact of hearing loss

Luc was diagnosed with severe hearing loss when he was in his early 20s. He wears a hearing aid and works as a postman in the Czech Republic. He finds the hearing aid seems to put people off talking to him and finds it difficult to make new friends. He doesn't go out much, for example to pubs or clubs, as he finds the background noise too difficult to handle. He lives on his own and feels really isolated. Most nights are spent watching TV with the subtitles or playing computer games. His doctor recommends he attends a lip-reading class and eventually he plucks up the courage to go. It is only through meeting other people with hearing loss that he starts to realise how depressed he has been feeling. Mixing with others in the same situation really helps him to

> (*Continued*)
>
> think about his own self-esteem and confidence and he realises he needs to take steps to address his feelings about losing his hearing.

> A hard of hearing or deafened client attending a health-related consultation may not only feel anxious about the health issue they are there to discuss, but on top of this may feel embarrassed about their hearing loss or the way their voice sounds and consequently the emotional impact of the hearing loss is likely to add another dimension to the healthcare consultation.

Within a hearing family, hearing children usually learn how to label their feelings and emotions through their voice and via spoken validation from their parents. However, deaf and hard of hearing children of hearing parents, who may struggle with communication, may have a delay in the acquisition of effective language. This in turn could play a part in delaying the development of emotional reasoning and the labelling of feelings together with the cognitive processes that accompany these (Henderson and Hendershott 1991 in Ralston and Israel 1995). This means that it may be more difficult for deaf and hard of hearing adults to express and describe their feelings and emotions than for a deaf child raised by deaf parents or a hearing child raised by hearing parents, who are less likely to have had the same communication difficulties.

The positive impact of having a family history of deafness

There is research evidence to indicate that deaf children of deaf parents fare better than deaf children of hearing parents in a number of different measures. For example, deaf children of deaf parents have fewer emotional and behavioural problems, better psychological functioning and fewer mental health issues compared to deaf children of hearing parents (Stephens 2005). As approximately 90% of deaf children are born to hearing parents there are evident issues for the large majority of deaf adults with congenital deafness.

Dafydd Stephens and Lesley Jones have edited a book '*The Impact of Genetic Hearing Impairment*' (2005), published by Whurr, which brings together a whole mixture of chapters that review the literature on the psychological impact of hearing loss on individuals; the reader is directed towards this for a more extensive overview.

Emotional issues to consider in a consultation

- Given the above, the adult who is deaf or hard of hearing who attends a healthcare consultation, whether they have been deaf from birth or whether they have lost their hearing as an adult, has a chance of being emotionally fragile and may have had to deal with difficult psychological issues throughout their lives.

- It is well known that deaf people generally have a much higher risk of mental health issues than hearing people (Department of Health 2005).

- It is vitally important that all health professionals involved use sensitive, empathic listening skills, make allowances for frustrations, do not respond negatively to seemingly overactive emotional responses to events and spend time to understand and support deaf and hard of hearing clients.

It is likely that deaf and hard of hearing people have previously had poor experiences of the health service, either through childhood or as an adult (as mentioned already in Chapter 2). This prior experience may mean that they come to a medical setting anticipating a poor service again and this may manifest as a defensive or aggressive stance. This will undoubtedly add to the emotional charge of a consultation.

When seeing a deaf client within a clinic setting consideration MUST be given to the potential for emotional fragility.

- If the health professional experiences a defensive stance from a deaf client it is important to view this with an empathic manner and to take care not to put additional stress on the client who is deaf, perhaps by overloading them with too much information.

- It can also help to use basic counselling skills, such as acknowledging openly some of the obvious difficulties; for example, by saying things like 'I can see you are really frustrated; however, I'm going to try really hard to understand what is going on for you' or 'I can understand that you are fed up with health professionals; help me to learn what I need to do to help you'.

- Emotional engagement within a healthcare consultation may be different for deaf and hard of hearing clients compared to hearing clients, although of course there are likely to be many exceptions and it is important not to over-generalise this. Any differences should also not be perceived as deficiencies, it is just a case of being aware and not surprised if differences exist.

Case study: taking it slowly

Kai is a deaf, Australian Sign Language (Auslan) user. He has had recurrent indigestion over a number of years and has been referred to an upper GI health professional to discuss having an exploratory endoscopy.

Kai has had a dreadful experience of the health service; he broke his leg when he was a teenager and was in hospital for a couple of months after having

(*Continued*)

complications post-surgery. None of his communication needs were met at the time, he had to struggle to lip-read what the doctors and nurses said to him and didn't understand most of what happened to him. This experience left him feeling angry and distrustful of all health professionals and he had avoided having anything to do with the health service since.

Kai arrived late for the consultation. A sign language interpreter had been booked and the upper GI nurse and interpreter have been waiting for him as he was the last appointment of the day. The nurse had deliberately structured her clinic in this way in case Kai had needed additional time.

The health professionals were aware that Kai might find the consultation difficult and so were mentally prepared to pay particular attention to his emotional needs. The clinic nurse went into the waiting room with the interpreter and asked his name and whether he would like to come into the consultation room. He looked sullen and unresponsive as he walked behind her into the room. As he slouched into his chair the nurse put her medical notes to one side, pulled her chair up in front of his and started with 'How are you?'

Kai signed that he hated hospitals and hoped that the consultation wouldn't take long. The nurse said, 'You can take as long as you need'. She said that the team were focussed on his needs; they wouldn't offer too much information in this first session but would use the time to take a full history and build a rapport between them. The nurse could see that Kai was suspicious and alienated and she knew that if she didn't give him the time and focus he needed it was unlikely he would engage with the service again.

Tinnitus

Tinnitus, or ringing in the ears, is incredibly common; in the UK one-third of adults have experienced this (Davis 1995). Tinnitus can occur in otherwise 'hearing' people but can also occur in people with hearing loss and deafness. People with a family history of deafness are thought to have a higher incidence of tinnitus and also a higher annoyance with this condition (Stephens, Lewis et al. 2003). Tinnitus is known to be incredibly distracting, can interfere with sleep and in some instances can severely affect quality of life.

Coping with tinnitus while also trying to cope with the information delivered in a healthcare setting (possibly also via an interpreter or communication support professional) can affect concentration enormously. Tinnitus can also become worse in times of stress. It is therefore vital that health professionals are particularly sensitive that this is an additional factor which may impact negatively on the exchange of communication. This is another reason why it is important to have more frequent, shorter consultations.

Post-clinic issues

As already discussed in Chapter 2, it is important to provide a choice of how post-clinic information is provided. Some deaf clients, particularly those who prefer to use speech, may be content to receive a written letter or leaflet summarising the take-home messages. As with all clients, deaf and hearing, this information should be adapted to the client's reading skills, should avoid jargon and be pitched appropriately.

Deaf sign language users may prefer to receive their post-clinic information in the form of a DVD in sign language. External companies are able to create such DVDs within a 24-hour turnaround, for a cost, and so this should not be difficult to organise. Research has shown that if a video or DVD is to be included that summarises a lot of health information, it is important to stick to a single health topic at a time. Too much information in one go can be confusing and difficult to process (Folkins, Sadler et al. 2005).

> Health professionals may need to adapt how they provide post-clinic information to deaf and hard of hearing clients. Long client letters with genetics jargon are unacceptable for both deaf sign users and hard of hearing speech users.

> Health professionals may need to translate client letters into plain English and/or an NSL on DVD.

Chapter 4

Specialist issues relevant to working with clients with neurofibromatosis Type 2

Wanda Neary

Overview of NF2

> For people with NF2 there are four major areas that impact on their lives (Neary, Stephens et al. 2006):
>
> - hearing difficulties
> - balance problems
> - facial weakness
> - difficulties with vision.

NF2 is a potentially life-threatening condition – the benign tumours in the head which cause the deafness may grow so large that they ultimately cut off brain function or the surgery to remove them may irreparably damage the brain. The combination of deafness with balance, visual, physical and psychological problems makes it very burdensome to some people. It is important for health professionals seeing clients with NF2 to have an awareness

Working with Deaf People – a Handbook for Health Professionals, ed. Anna Middleton. Published by Cambridge University Press. © Cambridge University Press 2010.

of the factors that can affect communication, in addition to the deafness.

- People with NF2 usually grow up being able to hear and use speech as their main form of communication.
- Clients are encouraged to lip-read as soon as they are diagnosed with NF2.
- Some clients are suitable for a cochlear implant, others will have an auditory brainstem implant inserted.
- A small percentage of clients and their families learn an NSL.
- Some people affected by NF2 have difficulties in that they do not feel part of the Hearing World because of their hearing problems, yet they do not automatically belong to the Deaf community as they usually cannot sign.
- A small number of clients with NF2 choose to have prenatal genetic diagnosis, with termination of pregnancy, to avoid transmitting the condition to their offspring.

> Health professionals should be sensitive to the psychological impact of NF2 as a potentially devastating disease for the affected individual and their family (Bance and Ramsden 1999 in Neary, Stephens et al. 2006).

- The health professional must ensure, as much as possible, that the client is prepared for the psychological blow of eventual total hearing loss and initiate appropriate training in non-auditory communication skills when necessary (Neary, Stephens et al. 2006).

- The impact is particularly marked in those families in which the disorder appears for the first time as a new mutation, and parental anxieties and guilt feelings are common (Neary, Stephens et al. 2006).

The person with NF2 may find a physical examination hard because of balance problems; this could mean that they find it awkward to climb onto an examination couch or hospital bed. The health professional should offer additional physical support to help with this.

The person with NF2 may have facial weakness and so be unable to speak clearly; they may also be very self-conscious of their speech and may not feel confident when they reply. The health professional needs to pay special attention to careful listening and be sensitive to feelings of discomfort.

The person with NF2 may find it difficult to read written notes because of dry-eye and visual problems. This may also mean that use of visual communication methods, such as lip-reading, use of a light-writer or note-taker, might be difficult. Providing written material in very large type may be helpful.

The Neurofibromatosis (NF) Association

In the UK there is a charity called the NF Association which provides support and information for people concerned about either NF1 or NF2. NF2 support workers are professionals employed by the charity who can visit individuals and their families affected by NF2 to offer practical and emotional support. They link in closely with health services.

A consultation in the specialist multidisciplinary NF2 clinic

The importance of multidisciplinary regional centres with experience in dealing with all aspects of NF2 has been emphasised (Evans, Baser et al. 2005), with input from neuro-otologists, neurosurgeons, ophthalmologists, geneticists, genetic counsellors, audiologists, speech therapists, counsellors, psychologists and occasionally psychiatrists being recommended. However, it is acknowledged that many hospitals do not offer this service yet and clients with NF2 are seen sporadically by different health professionals.

The following summarises what happens in a specialist NF2 clinic in Manchester, UK:

- The client's MRI scans will be carefully examined and reported on by the consultant neuroradiologist from the multidisciplinary NF2 team. The report and scans will be available for viewing by the client in clinic.

- No more than five clients will be booked for each clinic, to allow time for full discussion with each client.
- The hospital reception staff are aware of the NF2 clinic, and welcome the clients in the appropriate manner, being mindful of the likelihood of a significant hearing loss (see Chapter 3 for details on deaf awareness).
- The chair for the appropriate member of the multidisciplinary team is positioned so that the professional's face is clearly visible to the client.
- Some clients with NF2 have balance and mobility problems, and will arrive in a wheelchair. It is essential that wheelchair access is available to the clinic.
- It is particularly helpful if the NF2 support worker (usually from the NF Association in the UK) welcomes the NF2 client in the waiting room, introduces himself/herself and then leads the client into the consultation room. If the client is in a wheelchair, the NF2 support worker can push the wheelchair into the consultation room, ensuring that the client is placed appropriately. She/he can then sit next to him, and help to interpret for the client as necessary.

Computers should be available to aid communication – the health professional can type directly into these and the client can then read from the device. The computer may take the form of a laptop, desktop or light-writer. The light-writer is particularly useful for people with visual as well as hearing impairment. Text is seen in a single line in large type and machines are relatively cheap to buy and light to carry.

- If the client uses an NSL or SSSL, an appropriate interpreter must be present at the consultation.
- Each professional from the multidisciplinary team will introduce himself/ herself to the client, so that the client will understand their role in the team.
- Members of the multidisciplinary team are mindful of the devastating impact of the disclosure of the diagnosis of NF2, particularly in a young person with no family history of NF2.
- Members of the multidisciplinary team should be mindful of not having parallel conversations between themselves during the client's consultation, as this can be confusing for the client.
- Although it is necessary to allow adequate time for discussion, the consultation should not be too lengthy. It is important that the client is aware of the fact that he/ she will receive a copy of the clinic letter following the consultation, which will summarise what was said in the consultation.

> The client may require considerable emotional support following a new diagnosis. The NF2 support worker can provide a contact telephone number following the consultation, extending an invitation to be contacted whenever the client feels this is necessary.

- The client should be given contact details of other NF2 clients who have given their consent to being contacted.

- The client should be given website details of NF2 chat rooms.
- The client will be aware that he/she will be followed up by the multidisciplinary NF2 team on a lifelong basis.
- Voice-recognition software is being explored for use in the NF2 clinic (Belk, Evans et al. 2008). Here, when the clinician speaks, this is turned into written text that the patient can read.

Case study: the impact of NF2 on the family

Adam is a 35-year-old man, whose father is known to have NF2. Adam's father took early retirement on medical grounds because of his NF2, and is now profoundly deaf, and is troubled with balance problems. Adam's father has been under the care of a specialist multidisciplinary NF2 clinic for 10 years. He has undergone surgery on three occasions to remove both of his eighth-nerve tumours and one spinal tumour. His children have all been invited to the multidisciplinary team, and all three adult children have undergone MRI scans. Adam has been found to have small eighth-nerve tumours on both sides, but at present he does not have any symptoms. Adam's progress will continue to be monitored by the specialist multidisciplinary team.

Adam is married, and he and his wife are anxious to know the risks of passing on NF2 to their children.

(*Continued*)

The 50% chance of passing on the altered NF2 gene with every pregnancy is explained and prenatal genetic testing is offered.

Comment

In this instance, with a family history of NF2, Adam may have a mindful awareness of the possibility for the diagnosis of NF2 in himself. Although it may still be a shock to have a new diagnosis he may cope better psychologically because he already has some familiarity with the condition through his father. The specialist multidisciplinary team are able to monitor Adam closely and recognise and manage his symptoms of NF2 as they arise.

Case study: the burden of NF2

Jacob was diagnosed with NF2 15 years ago. There is a strong family history of NF2, with his mother and one of his three siblings being affected. Jacob has undergone surgery for both vestibular Schwannomas, and has no hearing. He took retirement on medical grounds 10 years ago. He has spinal tumours, and is confined to a wheelchair. He suffers from bilateral dry-eye, and has difficulties with his vision. He is cared for by his wife, Anna. They have four children, two of whom are known to have inherited the NF2 mutation. Jacob is reviewed by the specialist multidisciplinary team on an annual basis.

Jacob arrives at the clinic for his annual appointment. He is in his wheelchair and is accompanied by his wife. Jacob is not able to communicate without the help of his wife. Because of his visual problems, he finds lip-reading extremely difficult and he has difficulty in using a light-writer. Anna helps to answer the questions for her husband during the consultation, explaining the questions and answers as the consultation progresses.

Jacob and Anna are particularly distressed that two of their four children are affected by NF2. They spend time with the geneticist and genetic counsellor talking through their concerns. The NF2 support worker arranges to make a home visit after the clinic appointment.

Comment

This family has a heavy load to bear. Jacob is very disabled, and relies on his wife for assistance in everyday living. There is a supportive GP and the District Nurse visit twice weekly to assist with bathing. Jacob and Anna have grave concerns for the future of their affected children. Members of the multidisciplinary team need to be sensitive to the medical, surgical and emotional needs of Jacob and the

(*Continued*)

need that Anna has for support, practical advice and understanding. The NF2 support worker has an important role in supporting this family, where difficulties continue to increase.

Emotional issues

It must be understood that the confirmation of the diagnosis of a dominantly transmitted genetic condition can have a marked impact on a client with NF2. In families with a known history of NF2, there is prior knowledge of the condition and an awareness of a possible diagnosis (Neary, Stephens et al. 2006). However, in a young person with currently mild symptoms, the diagnosis and future implications may come as a dreadful, unexpected shock. Education may have to be cut short, and close personal relationships may sometimes be terminated. Previously organised career pathways may need to be abandoned. A working life may not be possible. Such individuals may need very considerable support from the professionals in charge of their care, their family and friends.

Professionals in charge of clients affected by NF2 should be sensitive to the likelihood of anxiety and depression in their clients (Neary, Stephens et al. 2006). The possibility of suicide should not be underestimated.

Case study: the value of a shared experience

Renata is a Polish woman of 45 years of age living in the UK. She has just received the diagnosis of NF2. She is accompanied by her husband. She had noted the sudden onset of right-sided tinnitus six months ago, and she felt that her right-sided hearing was down. There is no family history of deafness. An MRI scan carried out at her local hospital had indicated bilateral vestibular Schwannomas.

Renata and her husband were shocked at the diagnosis, and asked whether it was possible to contact another client already diagnosed with NF2. The NF2 support worker gave her the contact details of a client with NF2 (Moses), who had previously said that he would be willing to speak to clients with NF2 who were finding the diagnosis difficult to come to terms with. Renata contacted Moses and arranged to meet at his home. Renata and her husband found this meeting to be most helpful. Moses had been diagnosed 20 years previously, and was still working full-time, despite being profoundly deaf. He was knowledgeable and open about his condition, and was pleased to answer Renata's questions.

Comment

Clients with NF2 can obtain considerable support from already-diagnosed clients who are willing to be

(*Continued*)

contacted by the newly diagnosed clients. In the UK information and support are also available from the Neurofibromatosis Association as well as Hearing Concern Link, which provides written information and courses and advises about weekends where people with NF2 can meet up.

Chapter 5

Specialist issues relevant to working with clients with deafblindness

Kerstin Möller

As already mentioned in previous chapters, it is very unusual for people with deafblindness to have total deafness as well as total blindness. There is usually a degree of either or both hearing and sight. A person with deafblindness has to concentrate hard to gather cues via their residual sight or hearing; this is both demanding and also tiring. People with deafblindness may be dependent on others around them to provide information about the outside world.

The impact of visual loss

The accompanying photographs represent what it might be like for a person with normal sight to see a clinic room, versus what it might be like for someone with impaired visual acuity, for example caused by congenital rubella syndrome (CRS).

The level of visual impairment can vary depending on the reason for the sight problem. For example, only one or

Working with Deaf People – a Handbook for Health Professionals, ed. Anna Middleton. Published by Cambridge University Press. © Cambridge University Press 2010.

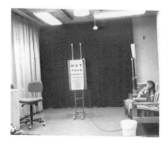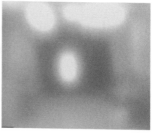

Left photograph represents normal visual acuity function 20/20 (1,0) and right photograph represents severe visual acuity impairment 20/1000 (0,020). Photographs courtesy of Göran Cedermark and Anders Hjälm, Ekeskolan.

both eyes might be affected or the vision difficulty might only apply in certain directions. A person with Usher syndrome aged 45–50 might only be able to see items that are in the centre of their line of sight, whereas a person with macular degeneration may only see what is at the periphery of their line of sight.

The brain will also fill in the gaps of what it is missing. For example, if the person with deafblindness is in a hospital canteen, they are expecting to see people, tables and chairs, food and drinks when they look around; however, a column in the room would be unexpected and so they might see this as something else (a piece of furniture, for example).

Information obtained in fragments increases the risk of misunderstanding. The more the individual has to strive to receive the message, the less capacity there is to understand the meaning of it.

The nature of the sight difficulties can vary enormously between individuals and also at different stages of life; therefore, in a clinic setting it is very important to ask the client to explain the nature of their specific situation.

A person with deafblindness will utilise the senses that they do have access to; this helps them receive information in ways different from those with sight and hearing.

> People with deafblindness who have limited sight and hearing will use other senses to help them gather information about their environment: for example, touch, smell and taste.

It is helpful if the health professional allows time at the beginning of a meeting with a person with deafblindness for the client to familiarise themselves with the health professional. This process may be done in several different ways and it is important for the health professional to not feel awkward about this or feel that it is not necessary; it is in fact vitally important for the person with deafblindness to use their senses to orientate themselves.

> Some clients with deafblindness may want to touch and feel the health professional's clothes (e.g. a collar or sleeve) or possibly feel the health professional's hair or face. Alternatively they may wish to sniff the air for perfume or smell the health professional's hand or cheek.

The process of using the remaining senses in a holistic manner and incorporating information gained from the environment is termed 'social haptic communication' (Lahtinen 2008) (see later for more detailed information).

> ### Case study: use of smell and support from 'haptics' in a consultation with someone who has early-onset deafblindness
>
> Sara is 15 years old and has CHARGE (see Chapter 2 for details). She lives in Switzerland. She has severe visual and hearing impairment as well as intellectual impairment. Sara uses tactile sign language to produce and receive signs in combination with speech.
>
> Sara is at the heart clinic for her annual follow-up, which involves having an echocardiogram (ECG). As part of the health professional's introduction to Sara the nurse offers her hand for Sara to shake; Sara also sniffs the hand so that she can gain a familiarity with the nurse. When the nurse goes to get the equipment to perform the ECG, she walks her fingers down Sara's arm, loses contact briefly so that she can bring the equipment closer, and then regains contact with Sara's arm and allows Sara to sniff her hand again so that Sara knows it is the same person. The nurse then gives one of the ECG electrodes to Sara and lets her examine it with her hands. Sara

remembers this procedure from the year before
and now that the introduction is over she is familiar
with what is going to happen and what is expected of
her; she removes her blouse so that the electrodes
can be attached.

Communication issues with deafblind clients

People with deafblindness can use several different ways
of communicating: this can range from gesture and
animation through to speech or variations in sign
language. An individual's expressive language, such as
spoken or signed, may remain unchanged throughout
their lifetime, but the methods of receiving information
could change many times during the individual's life.
For example, a person who develops hearing loss first
while their sight is good may learn to communicate
using visual sign language and use this as their first or
preferred language (in the same way as a person who
has just deafness on its own might). Later, when their
sight gets worse, they may adapt their visual sign
language to tactile sign language, which enables the
person to put their hand on top of the hand of a person
who is signing. The shape and position of the hands
deliver the language.

This is in contrast to a deafblind person who has
relatively good hearing to start with, but it is their sight that
is restricted. They may use speech, hearing and Braille as

their primary mode of communication. Later when their hearing deteriorates they may move to Braille and tactile sign language that utilises finger-spelling. They may also continue to use speech too even though they can no longer hear effectively.

Some people with deafblindness are educated at university level whereas others have fragmentary general knowledge, restricted by their difficulties in accessing the world. There are also people with deafblindness who communicate at a level considered 'pre-language' and also those who express themselves without intent.

The ability to communicate is largely affected by whether there are associated learning difficulties in conjunction with the sensory impairments. In addition to this, some people who are deafblind have their visual and hearing impairments from birth and therefore before language would have developed naturally. They will still communicate, but the way they do this may only be understood by the people closest to them. For such people it is important to ask the caregivers the most appropriate way to communicate.

> One of the first steps in establishing effective communication with someone who has deafblindness is to find out first what is their preferred language and mode of communication and to work with this.

Case study: adapting communication style

Mr Brown is in his 80s and has got macular degeneration. He lives in Jamaica; he has also been losing his hearing since he was in his 50s. He recently developed a pain in his groin and has been referred to a prostate cancer clinic. This is his first visit to the clinic and he is unsure where to go. The map that he has been sent is too small for him to read. The receptionist tries without success to tell him where to go and shows him on the map. He starts to feel frustrated that he cannot see what she is pointing to and also cannot hear what she is saying. She recognises that he is becoming confused with the information and realises that she will have to adapt how she communicates. She takes out a yellow sheet of paper and draws in thick pen on it. She writes, **GO STRAIGHT DOWN CORRIDOR, CLINIC FIRST LEFT.** Mr Brown is delighted: he can clearly see the instructions, his frustration disappears and he regains his confidence. He walks over to the clinic by himself, pleased that he was able to receive the support he needed.

Recommendations for the clinic

Given the enormous effort it takes for a person with deafblindness to use their residual hearing and sight to make sense of the information around them, it is usual

> (*Continued*)
>
> in a clinic setting to allow recognition of this by planning both short breaks (less than 1 minute) and longer breaks (from 5 minutes to an hour). It is also helpful to plan for multiple consultations if necessary rather than trying to fit too much information into one.

When the brain is working hard to receive information it will often fill in the gaps when information is partial or missing. It is therefore vital to deliver information in several different ways and to check understanding frequently.

Conversing with a person with visual impairment can be helped by a few simple steps. For example, jewellery that glitters can be very distracting; when it catches the light this can give confusing visual cues to the person with restricted vision. It is also helpful to have a consultation in a room where the light doesn't continually vary, for example, alternating sunlight and shade through a window with no curtain. Curtains that screen out variations in light intensity can be very helpful. Women who wear lipstick can also be more easily seen than those who do not.

It is very important for the deafblind client's medical records to be clearly marked with their communication requirements; for example, on the front page of the notes there could be three bullet points which say:

- Uses visual sign language
- Slower tempo needed
- Written materials, yellow paper, Arial 16 point

These reminders need to be clear and easily accessible for the health professional and should also be checked and updated regularly as it is likely that the client's needs will change over time as their condition progresses.

The physical environment

Some people with deafblindness are more sensitive to light than others. Both those with Alström syndrome and those with Usher syndrome have retinitis pigmentosa, which causes impaired night blindness, impaired adaptability to light as well as impaired contrast sensitivity. Youngsters with Usher syndrome may be dazzled by a white sheet of paper, a white tablecloth or even the glass on the front of a painting. Youngsters with Alström have, in general, lost virtually all of their sight, while an elderly person with Usher syndrome is likely to still have some residual sight.

Other people with deafblindness who have residual visual function left need good levels of light in order to be able to utilise the sight that they do have. For example, dimly lit rooms can make it difficult to see. This means it is vitally important to ask clients what their preferences and needs are and to make attempts to address these. What is most helpful within the clinic setting is to have the flexibility to alter the environment as necessary.

The environment surrounding the clinic setting also needs to be considered. For example, steps, banisters and columns should be clearly marked and this can be done by using contrasting colours. It is best to do this at a new building stage; however, it is still possible to make improvements to existing structures.

> Some suggestions for improving the environment include adding a large colour print to a white column, winding long pieces of coloured cloth around a white banister and painting steps so that they are clearly defined. Signs also need to be considered, using large, blocked, yellow writing on a coloured background.

Consideration can also be given to the clothes that the health professional wears. For example, a white coat is likely to dazzle a person with retinitis pigmentosa; a large wristwatch or jewellery could also be covered.

> For people who receive sign language visually it is important that there is good contrast between the clothes of the signer and the colour of their skin.

Case study: consideration for practical aspects of the clinic with a deafblind client

Stefan is 45 years old and has Usher syndrome type II. He lives in Denmark. He cannot hear speech in a noisy environment and has progressive visual impairment. At the moment he has some sight but is bothered by direct light (such as sunshine) and is easily dazzled, for example by jewellery that catches the light or by light sporadically flitting into a room through window blinds.

Stefan goes to see his GP. The GP practice has made a specific effort to address the needs of their clients with deafblindness. The waiting room has undergone acoustic analysis and the echo has been adjusted. The windows have curtains that reduce light variation. The light in the waiting room is indirect and soft. The reception staff have a simple dress code, with no sparkly jewellery or name badges that can reflect the light. They are also allowed to wear lipstick if they choose. They use a clear voice when speaking to deafblind clients and always ask their clients whether they prefer to be escorted into the GP's room. The GP also knows that if he/she needs to remove Stefan's glasses or hearing aids for an examination they will always tell Stefan where they have been put. Stefan's medical records clearly state his needs from a communication sense so it is easy for the GP to prepare.

Comments

Another person with the same diagnosis may not have the same requirements and Stefan's preferences shift according to progression of his visual and hearing impairment. Therefore the communication recommendations in his record need to be often updated.

Conversing in speech with someone who has deafblindness

- When conversing with a deafblind person many of the same deaf awareness skills, as discussed in Chapter 2, can be applied. It is not necessary to speak louder or exaggerate lip-patterns; however, it may be helpful to slow the tempo slightly. It is also helpful to face the person, speak clearly and apply all the techniques to support lip-reading.
- It is also important to avoid having a consultation with lots of background noise, e.g. from a waiting room or busy corridor.

Conversing in visual sign language with someone who has deafblindness

- Sign language is a very visual language, therefore if someone who uses sign language loses some of their vision then this can impact enormously on their ability to communicate.
- The degree of difficulty in using sign language is impacted upon by the level and nature of the vision problems. For example, some of the signs or the positioning of them may be hidden due to a vision blind spot. Alternatively, field vision restrictions may make it more difficult to see signs outside certain parameters.
- Vision restrictions that affect the ability to determine differences in contrast will also affect the ability to

receive sign language. For example, if the person with deafblindness is conversing with a signer who has pale skin, pale clothing and little contrasting colours on them then this may make it difficult for a person with retinitis pigmentosa to see.

- A person with Usher syndrome may need to step back in order to receive a broader view of the person signing.
- Conversely others with deafblindness may need to be extremely close to the signer in order to be able to see what is being signed.

> It is very important for the health professional to ask the person with deafblindness what the most appropriate distance is for them to be sitting. The distance between the health professional and the person with deafblindness will need to be negotiated as it will vary from person to person.

- A person signing can help someone with deafblindness by wearing contrasting colours, e.g. dark skin – light clothing or vice versa.

Conversing in tactile sign language with someone who has deafblindness

- A conversation in tactile sign language requires the 'producer' (person 'talking') and 'receiver' (person 'listening') to have contact with each other via their hands.

- The producing hand is underneath and the receiving hand is on top of this following what the person is signing. When a change-over happens with respect to the person leading the conversation, the hands swap over so that the receiver becomes the producer.
- Tactile sign language is based on visual sign language, but all the expression that would have been seen in the signer's face is translated to their hands.
- The optimal seating arrangements in tactile sign language vary from person to person; some people like to sit or stand opposite their conversation partner. Other people prefer to sit side by side.

Skilled tactile sign language users can talk with one hand and listen with the other.

- There are several methods of tactile sign language. This can be a more complete language as in visual sign language (an NSL) or could be just constructed of finger-spelt words. For this latter method one can use letters of the alphabet that are derived from sign language letters or from written letters and these can be delivered to the receiver on their palm or even forehead.
- Different parts of the palm can denote different letters.
- Alternatively, the receiver may put their hand at the throat of a person who is talking and feel the vibrations of what is being said.

- A hearing/sighted person who wants to communicate with someone who has deafblindness needs to think carefully and sensitively about how to do this. An important point is not to frighten or startle the person with deafblindness by suddenly taking their hand or physically moving them without previous discussion.

An introduction can be made through a gentle touch on the arm; this alerts the person with deafblindness that there is someone new who wishes to converse with them. It may be helpful to gently give something to the person with deafblindness that can help them to identify who wishes to communicate; for example, a doctor might hand over a stethoscope to feel.

Case study: conversation between someone with deafblindness and a health professional who does not know how to use tactile sign language

Allen is 55 years old and has Usher syndrome type I. He can hardly hear anything and he has very little vision in the centre-left of his field. Allen lives in Denmark and has gone to his local Emergency department because he has fallen over and hurt his foot.

When he arrives in the Emergency room at the hospital his left foot is very painful, swollen and red. The health professionals see immediately that he has deafblindness and so call for an on-site interpreter.

(*Continued*)

While they are waiting for the interpreter, the doctor arrives and wants to introduce herself to Allen.

The doctor gently touches Allen's right arm. When Allen gives his hand the doctor puts her stethoscope in it. Allen understands that this person is the doctor and the two of them shake hands. Allen points to his swollen foot and indicates that it is hurting. The doctor touches the other foot and gently presses it. She is indicating to Allen that she needs to examine his swollen foot but before she touches the wounded foot she wants to forewarn Allen of what she needs to do. She waits for Allen to indicate that it is OK for her to proceed in touching his normal foot. In order to show him what the examination will be like, she then pushes the normal foot and bends it in several directions; she then touches his wounded foot and waits. She looks to see whether Allen gives an indication that it is all right for her to proceed. He nods at her and so she picks up the wounded foot and presses and bends it in the same way; it is very painful but Allen is prepared and feels secure that the doctor is doing what is necessary. The doctor thinks that Allen ought to have an X-ray but she doesn't know how to pass this message to Allen. However, at this moment the interpreter arrives.

Comment

Even though the doctor in this scenario had no knowledge of how to use tactile sign language, this did not preclude her from communicating effectively with Allen. She was very courteous and respectful of Allen and his physical space. She did not invade it without first checking with him that this was all right and took her time to demonstrate what she needed to do.

Using written language to communicate

Many people with deafblindness have an ability to read and write, although if the deafness developed very early on and before the vision loss, then this may not necessarily be the case if sign language is the preferred language. If there is written language, then it is possible to communicate using this in a variety of different ways. The writing could be done on a computer, on paper or on the deafblind person's hand. Consideration will usually need to be given to the size, shape and colour of the letters as well as the background colour.

- For people with impaired visual acuity, increase the size of text and use block letters rather than a handwriting typeface.
- For people with macular degeneration use thick text, e.g. written with a felt-tipped pen rather than biro, or in bold rather than regular type.
- For people with impaired colour vision use black letters instead of red or blue.

On a computer, Arial or Verdana are usually easier to read than Times New Roman or italics. Also, start with typeface size 14 and increase as necessary. Using a dark blue background to the page and yellow lettering can also help. Note that pictures should be accompanied by textual commentary.

Using Braille to communicate

Braille can be used by marking out the Braille letters on a hand or using equipment which the sighted person can type messages into, e.g. Tellatouch, Versabraille; the person with deafblindness receives these messages on their fingers through a small Braille screen. The person with deafblindness can then type a Braille message and it is converted into written text for the sighted person to read.

Some people with deafblindness use a mobile Braille reader. This can be used with an adapted mobile telephone to receive and send messages. It is also possible to connect these to a computer keyboard: the hearing/sighted person writes into the keyboard and this is converted into a Braille message for the person with deafblindness.

Social-haptic communication

Recently, a form of communication called the 'social-haptic communication system' has been defined which many people with deafblindness use (Lahtinen 2008). In 'social-haptics' the body and senses are used together to produce and receive information. This is a form of communication that relies not on the construction of language but more on the experience gained from touch (as well as smell and taste for people with deafblindness). For example, body drawing and physical contact between people offer a form of communication that has no sentence construction or words, but allows an exchange of information that can result in an expression of feelings and emotions. The use of guiding (where a sighted person directs a visually impaired person in a particular way) as well as physically interacting with each other (e.g. via stroking, pinching or tickling) is a classic form of social-haptic communication. Social-haptics are often discussed in relation to the creation of art through movement.

Dealing with a progressive loss of ability

When a person has an impairment that progressively gets worse they have to frequently adapt to new ways of coping. A decrease in the ability to receive information from the outside world through sight and hearing requires a change in cognition and this can be accompanied by an upheaval of emotions. First, the person may find it difficult to carry on with the old ways of coping and may also feel a sense of loss that they cannot continue as they did before but have to adapt how they communicate. For example, a sign language user may find it incredibly difficult to accept that they are no longer coping in visual sign language alone; perhaps their vision has deteriorated to a level where they are now unable to see most of a conversation and they need to start learning tactile sign language. Second, having to continually relearn and cope with decreasing levels of sight and hearing is very tiring. Tiredness in itself may affect the ability to see and hear.

Interpreters for people with deafblindness

- It is often very helpful for interpreters and health professionals to have a pre-clinic conversation prior to the consultation with the deafblind client, so that the interpreter can be briefed on what the health professional plans to discuss. This is the same for consultations with deaf patients, as discussed in Chapter 2.
- The aim of the pre-clinic discussion is so that the interpreter can prepare the way that they will translate the conversation and can also clarify the meaning of medical concepts that will be used.
- If the heath professional is planning on doing a physical examination then it is also helpful to discuss this generally so that the interpreter can plan how this will be explained to the client.

> Interpreters for clients with deafblindness are slightly different from interpreters for deaf clients in that they not only interpret the spoken word, but also interpret visual information, as well as guiding the deafblind client, e.g. leading them into the consultation room on their arm.

- There are a number of different ways that a consultation may be interpreted between a speaking health professional and a deafblind client:
  - From speech to visual or tactile sign language
  - From speech to clearer speech
  - From speech to writing
- The interpreter will also provide information on the visual setting, e.g. describing the environment, people, events, social interplay, atmosphere
- The interpreter will 'guide' the client: this is a physical support which helps the client when walking or in transportation and often involves the interpreter offering their arm for the client to touch as they walk

Case study: interpreting for several deafblind people at once

A meeting is happening at a hospital in Sweden between staff at the eye clinic and four delegates from the local branch of the deafblind association.

(*Continued*)

The meeting is arranged to discuss the restoration of the waiting room in the clinic. There are eight professional deafblind interpreters booked for this event (two per deafblind client). One is operating while the other is in a supporting position and every five minutes they swap roles.

Lily uses tactile sign language. Eve uses tactile signs with finger-spelt letters based on Swedish letters and grammar. Ken uses visual sign language with adjustments made to account for his requirements of light and distance. Glen uses written interpretation.

Ken is the most dependent on getting the light adjusted in the room so that he can make the most of his visual skills; he also needs to position his interpreter at a particular distance from him so that he can optimise the vision he has. Therefore, no one takes a seat until Ken and his interpreters have worked out the optimal positioning. The interpreters working with Ken are labelled the 'central interpreters'. Behind these interpreters a dark green cloth is put up on the white wall so as to minimise the glare from the whiteness of the wall.

Lily is seated with her two interpreters beside her. She can receive tactile sign language on her left as well as her right hand. She receives the signs via the interpreter's hand, which moves in a certain spatial position to convey language. One of the interpreters, however, can only produce tactile sign language fast with her right hand. Therefore these two interpreters shift place from time to time. One is operating while the other is supporting.

Eve is placed with her back to Ken; this means that 'her' interpreters are visually opposite the central interpreters and thus can see what they are discussing (and are therefore able to interpret this). Eve is using tactile signing based on finger-spelling, but this is different from the signing that Lily is using.

Glen and the writing interpreters sit together: these interpreters write their interpretation into a computer and the large text appears on a screen that he can see. The screen is also adjusted specifically to the correct distance and colour for Glen.

When each person wants to say something this is interpreted for the other three deafblind people by their own individual interpreters. When Lily wants to say something, she stands in front of the green cloth and uses sign language. When Glen says something it is interpreted into sign language by the central interpreters.

Staff from the eye clinic sit around the room. They have provided two maps of the proposed waiting room for the deafblind delegates to discuss. One is a tactile map; Lily and Eve scrutinise this using their fingers. The other is a visual drawing, which has been enlarged and is hung on the wall; Ken and Glen look at this. Whenever Lily and Eve want to walk around the room they use guiding the whole time. When Ken goes to

(*Continued*)

look at the map, he uses guiding but Glen prefers to go by himself.

Lily, Eve and their interpreters all needed chairs without armrests so that they could use tactile sign language freely, therefore these specific chairs were reserved for them.

Identity and emotional issues

Health education in the emotional aspects of deafblindness is very important if a holistic approach is to be taken in caring for this group of people. A deafblind person constantly receives fragmentary information; this makes it difficult to trust what is being seen or heard. This means that they can feel vulnerable and also very exposed (Möller 2008); in addition to this they are also known to experience ontological insecurity (Danermark and Möller 2008).

It is therefore usual for someone with deafblindness to relentlessly question whether they accurately understand their environment. This can, in turn, affect their self-image, self-esteem and confidence. Deafblind people often feel incredibly vulnerable. Skilled, interdisciplinary social and health workers are usually a large part of a deafblind person's life.

Case study: growing up with deafblindness

Rose from Sweden is 50 years old. She has Usher syndrome type I; she has total hearing impairment and a very severe visual impairment. She has grown up using visual sign language as her first language and has many Deaf friends. She tells the social worker at the Deafblind Rehabilitation Centre about her childhood.

Rose started school aged 7 years and at that time had no language at all: she had been deaf prelingually and had not been taught sign language or speech. She calls the years where she had no language 'the white years'. Her parents were encouraged to teach her speech and her mother tried hard but it was very difficult because Rose had never heard sound.

Rose was sent to a boarding school for deaf children. In the beginning she was terrified because she didn't understand what was happening but gradually she was introduced to sign language. The children at the school were not allowed to sign in class but in the school breaks and out of school this was the language they used. Rose was gradually introduced to the Deaf community and therefore to sign language. For the first time in her life, she felt that she belonged somewhere and she had friends with whom she could easily communicate.

While her sight was relatively good, Rose developed into a confident member of the Deaf community and attended her local Deaf club

(Continued)

regularly. However, more recently her sight has deteriorated and she can no longer see visual sign language. Rose says that nowadays she sits at home and no longer goes out. She has withdrawn from the Deaf community and no longer goes to the Deaf club as she can't participate in signed conversations. Rose can still use the computer (the text is presented in large, clear type) and keeps in contact with her friends via email.

Comments

Withdrawal from social contact is a common strategy for people who gradually lose their sight and/or hearing. Rose would benefit enormously from interacting with deafblind services that can help her develop tactile sign language and other forms of communication. Her confidence has also dropped since she can no longer see visual sign language. She is a prime candidate for depression and the deafblind services who support her will be very aware of helping her deal with this.

Research has shown that youngsters with deafblindness have sometimes experienced lack of consideration from people they interact with; they also report that at times they have felt denigrated or insulted (Möller and

Danermark 2007). It is known that if support and information is offered to those who surround people with deafblindness it is possible to improve the social interaction between them (Mar and Sall 1995).

> Visual impairments are particularly traumatic to Deaf people and there is often a very real phobia about developing blindness (Cioffi 1996).

- Social withdrawal is a very common coping mechanism for people with deafblindness.
- Withdrawal by people with early-onset deafblindness may be misinterpreted as autism.
- Denial is another strategy, where people refuse to walk with a white stick, guide or guide dog, in spite of obvious needs.
- Promiscuity has also been shown in some people with deafblindness and is thought to be a result of difficulties in dealing with grief and pain due to the increasing levels of disability (Fillman, Leguire et al. 1989, Vernon and Andrews 1990).
- Self-harm and repetitive habits are also ways of expressing frustration and inability to cope with the implications of an early-onset deafblindness.
- The above behaviour can be addressed when the social environment around a deafblind person improves, consisting of interaction with people who understand how to work with persons who have deafblindness (Janssen, Riksen-Walraven et al. 2004).

Useful website addresses

The websites that have been consulted in the preparation of this book are listed below:

Charities and support groups

The International Federation of the Hard of Hearing
  http://www.ifhoh.org
World Federation of the Deaf
  http://www.wfdeaf.org/
Royal National Institute for Deaf People
  http://www.rnid.org.uk/
British Deaf Association
  http://bda.org.uk/
National Deaf Children's Society
  http://www.ndcs.org.uk/
Hearing Concern Link
  http://www.hearingconcernlink.org
Hearing Dogs for Deaf People
  http://www.hearingdogs.org.uk
The Guide Dogs for the Blind Association
  http://www.guidedogs.org.uk

Neurofibromatosis Association
  http://www.nfauk.org
Nordic Centre for Welfare and Social Issues
  http://www.nud.dk
The Information Centre for Acquired Deafblindness
  (in Denmark)
  http://www.dbcent.dk/vcfdbb/subpage19.aspx
Deafblind International
  http://www.deafblindinternational.org/standard/
    conferences.html
Sense for deafblind people
  http://www.sense.org.uk
Helen Keller National Center for Deaf-Blind Youths
  and Adults
  http://www.hknc.org
The World Federation of the Deafblind
  http://www.wfdb.org
CHARGE syndrome
  http://www.chargesyndrome.org/about-charge.asp
Congenital rubella syndrome
  http://www.hknc.org/Rubella.htm

Companies that will translate written material into plain English or BSL

TeamHado: http://www.teamhado.com
EyeGaze: http://www.eyegaze.tv/cm/
AC2.com: http://www.ac2.com/
Remark!: http://www.remark.uk.com/

Companies that offer deaf awareness training and deaf equality training

Deafworks: http://www.deafworks.co.uk/
Sense-Ability: http://www.sense-ability.co.uk
RNID: http://www.rnid.org.uk
Deaf Aware: http://www.deafaware.com/

Companies that offer live, on-line interpreting in BSL

Sign Translate: http://www.signtranslate.com (which also allows access to a list of predefined medical questions with an immediate BSL translation)
Sign Video: http://www.signvideo.co.uk

Miscellaneous

Equality and Human Rights Commission: http://www.equalityhumanrights.com

– good information on applying the DDA in practice

Gene Clinics: http://www.geneclinics.org

– overview of deafness, genetics and management

University of Manchester webpages on genetic counselling in sign language: http://sites.mhs.manchester.ac.uk/what-is-genetic-counselling/

APPENDIX

Diagnostic criteria for NF2

- Diagnostic criteria for NF2 were agreed by the NIH Consensus Development Conference on Neurofibromatosis in 1987 and additional criteria were described by Evans et al. in 1992 to allow for the diagnosis of NF2 in individuals affected with multiple intracranial and spinal tumours, but not bilateral vestibular Schwannomas.

Table 1 Diagnostic criteria for NF2

A diagnosis of NF2 is made in a client who has:

• Bilateral vestibular Schwannomas

Or

• A family history of NF2

Plus

• A unilateral vestibular Schwannoma

Or any two of:

• Meningioma, glioma, neurofibroma, Schwannoma, posterior subcapsular lenticular opacities

(NIH 1987)

(*Continued*)

A diagnosis of NF2 is made in a client who has:

• A unilateral vestibular Schwannoma

Plus any two of:

• Meningioma, glioma, neurofibroma, Schwannoma, posterior subcapsular lenticular opacities

Or

• Multiple meningiomas (two or more)

(Evans, Huson et al. 1992b)

REFERENCES

Arnos, K. S., J. Israel, et al. (1991). Genetic counselling for the deaf: medical and cultural considerations. *Annals of the New York Academy of Sciences,* **630**, 212–22.

Arnos, K. S., J. Israel, et al. (1992). Genetic counselling for the deaf. *Otolaryngologic Clinics of North America,* **25**(5), 953–71.

Bance, M. and R. Ramsden (1999). Management of neurofibromatosis type 2. *Ear Nose and Throat Journal,* **78**, 91–4.

Barnett, S. (2002a). Communication with deaf and hard of hearing people: a guide for medical education. *Academic Medicine,* **77**(7), 694–700.

Barnett, S. (2002b). Cross-cultural communication with patients who use American Sign Language. *Family Medicine,* **34**, 376–82.

Barnett, S. (2002c). *Deafblind Culture.* Bristol: University of Bristol Centre for Deaf Studies.

Belk, R. (2006). Seeing chromosomes: improving access to culturally sensitive genetic counselling through the provision of genetic information in British Sign Language. In D. Stephens and L. Jones, eds. *The Effects of*

Genetic Hearing Impairment in the Family. Chichester: Wiley, pp. 285–96.

Belk, R., D. Evans, et al. (2008). Evaluation of voice recognition software supporting communication with deafened people in the Neurofibromatosis type 2 (Nf2) clinic. British Society of Human Genetics Conference, York. *Journal of Medical Genetics,* **45**, S09.

Belk, R. and A. Middleton (2004). Seeing chromosomes – translating genetic information into British Sign Language. European Psychosocial Aspects of Genetics Conference, Munich. *European Journal of Human Genetics,* **12**, Suppl. 1.

Bell, A. (1883). Upon the formation of a deaf variety of the human race. *National Academy of Sciences Memoirs,* **2**, 177–262.

Biesold, H. (1999). *Crying Hands: Eugenics and Deaf People in Nazi Germany.* Washington DC: Gallaudet University Press.

British Deaf Association (2005). Factsheet on using a sign language interpreter. London, British Deaf Association in-house publication.

Campbell, R., M. MacSweeney, et al. (2008). Sign language and the brain: a review. *Journal of Deaf Studies and Deaf Education,* **13**(1 Winter), 3–20.

Cioffi, J. (1996). Orientation and mobility and the Usher syndrome client. *Journal of Vocational Rehabilitation,* **6**(2), 175–83.

Cohen, M. and R. Gorlin (1995). Epidemiology, etiology and genetic patterns. In R. Gorlin, H. Toriello and

M. Cohen, eds. *Hereditary Hearing Loss and Its Syndromes.* New York: Oxford University Press.

Danermark, B. and K. Möller (2008). Deafblindness, ontological security, and social recognition. *International Journal of Audiology,* **47**(Suppl 2), 119–23.

Davis, A. (1995). *Hearing in Adults.* London: Whurr.

Davis, A. C. (1989). The prevalence of hearing impairment and reported hearing disability among adults in Great Britain. *International Journal of Epidemiology,* **18**(4), 911–17.

Department of Health (2005). *Mental Health and Deafness: Towards Equity and Access. Best Practice Guidelines.* Avavilable from http://www.dh.gov.uk/en/Publicationsandstatistics/Publications/PublicationsPolicyAndGuidance/DH_4103995 [Accessed 16 Feb 08].

Dolnick, E. (1993). Deafness as culture. *The Atlantic Monthly,* **272**(3), 37–53.

Dye, M. and J. Kyle (2001). *Deaf People in the Community: Health and Disability.* Bristol: Deaf Studies Trust, pp. 1–135.

Erting, C. (1994). *Deafness, Communication, Social Identity: Ethnography in a Pre-School for Deaf Children.* Burtonsville, MD: Linstock Press.

Estivill, X., P. Fortina, et al. (1998). Connexin-26 mutations in sporadic and inherited sensorineural deafness. *Lancet,* **351**, 394–8.

Evans, D., M. Baser, et al. (2005). Management of the client and family with neurofibromatosis 2: a consensus conference statement. *British Journal of Neurosurgery,* **19**(1), 5–12.

Evans, D., J. Birch, et al. (1999). Paediatric presentation of Type 2 Neurofibromatosis. *Archives of Disease in Childhood,* **81**, 496–9.

Evans, D., S. Huson, et al. (1992a). A genetic study of type 2 neurofibromatosis in the United Kingdom. 1. Prevalence, mutation rate, fitness and confirmation of maternal transmission effect on severity. *Journal of Medical Genetics,* **29**, 841–6.

Evans, D., S. Huson, et al. (1992b). A genetic study of type 2 neurofibromatosis in the United Kingdom. 2. Guidelines for genetic counselling. *Journal of Medical Genetics,* **29**, 847–52.

Fillman, R., L. Leguire, et al. (1989). Consideration for serving adolescents with Usher's syndrome. *Review Rehabilitation and Education for Blindness and Visual Impairment,* **21**(1), 19–25.

Firth, H. V. and J. A. Hurst (2005). *Oxford Desk Reference: Clinical Genetics.* Oxford: Oxford University Press.

Fischer, S. D. and H. Van der Hulst (2003). Sign language structures. In M. Marschark and P. E. Spencer, eds. *Oxford Handbook of Deaf Studies, Language and Education.* Oxford: Oxford University Press, pp. 319–31.

Folkins, A., G. R. Sadler, et al. (2005). Improving the Deaf community's access to prostate and testicular cancer information: a survey study. *BioMed Central Public Health,* **5**(63).

Fortnum, H., G. Barton, et al. (2006). The impact for children of having a family history of hearing impairment in a UK-wide population study. In D. Stephens and L. Jones, eds. *The Effects of Genetic Hearing Impairment in the Family.* Chichester: Wiley, pp. 29–42.

Gibson, I. (2004). Summary: Teaching strategies used to develop short-term memory in deaf children. *Deafness and Education International,* **6**(3), 171–2.

Grundfast, K. M. and J. Rosen (1992). Ethical and cultural considerations in research on hereditary deafness. *Otolaryngologic Clinics of North America,* **25**(5), 973–8.

Harkins, J. E. and M. Bakke (2003). Technologies for communication: status and trends. In M. Marschark and P. E. Spencer, eds. *Oxford Handbook of Deaf Studies, Language and Education.* Oxford: Oxford University Press, pp. 406–19.

Harmer, L. M. (1999). Health care delivery and deaf people: practice, problems, and recommendations for change. *Journal of Deaf Studies and Deaf Education,* **4**(2), 73–110.

Hartong, D., E. Berson, et al. (2006). Retinitis pigmentosa. *The Lancet,* **368**(9549), 1795–809.

Henderson, D. and A. Hendershott (1991). ASL and the family system. *American Annals of the Deaf,* **136**(4), 325–9.

Hilgert, N., R. Smith, et al. (2008). Forty-six genes causing nonsyndromic hearing impairment: Which ones should be analyzed in DNA diagnostics. *Mutation Research* [Epub ahead of print].

Hoffmeister, R. (1985). Families with deaf parents: a functional perspective. In S. K. Thurman, ed. *Children of*

Handicapped Parents: Research and Clinical Perspectives. Orlando, FL: Academic Press, pp. 111–30.

Iezzoni, L. I., B. L. O'Day, et al. (2004). Communicating about health care: observations from persons who are deaf or hard of hearing. *Annals of Internal Medicine,* **140**, 356–62.

Israel, J., Ed. (1995). *An Introduction to Deafness: A Manual for Genetic Counselors.* Washington DC: Genetic Services Center, Gallaudet University.

Israel, J. and K. Arnos (1995). Genetic evaluation and counseling strategies: the genetic services center experience. In J. Israel, ed. *An Introduction to Deafness: A Manual for Genetic Counselors.* Washington DC: Genetic Services Center, Gallaudet University, pp. 181–208.

Janssen, M., J. Riksen-Walraven, et al. (2004). Enhancing the interactive competence of deafblind children: do intervention effects endure? *Journal of Developmental and Physical Disabilities,* **16**(1), 73–95.

Kaplan, H., S. Bally, et al. (1987). *Speechreading: A Way to Improve Understanding.* Washington DC: Gallaudet University Press.

Kaplan, H., V. Gladstone, et al. (1993). *Audiometric Interpretation: A Manual of Basic Audiometry.* Boston: Allyn and Bacon.

Kelley, P. M., D. J. Harris, et al. (1998). Novel mutations in the connexin 26 gene (GJB2) that cause autosomal recessive (DFNB1) hearing loss. *American Journal of Human Genetics,* **62**, 792–9.

Kimberling, W. and C. Möller (1995). Clinical and molecular genetics of Usher syndrome. *Journal of the American Academy of Audiology,* **6**, 63–72.

Kleinig, D. and H. Mohay (1991). A comparison of the health knowledge of hearing-impaired and hearing high school students. *American Annals of the Deaf,* **135**(3), 246–51.

Ladd, P. (1988). The modern Deaf community. In S. Gregory and G. Hartley, eds. *Constructing Deafness.* London: Open University Press, pp. 35–9.

Ladd, P. (2003). *Understanding Deaf Culture: In Search of Deafhood.* Clevedon, UK: Multilingual Matters.

Lahtinen, R. (2008). *Haptices and Haptemes (A Case Study of Developmental Process in Social-Haptic Communication of Acquired Deafblind People).* Frinton on Sea: A1 Management UK.

Lass, L., R. Franklin, et al. (1978). Health knowledge, attitudes and practices of the deaf population in Greater New Orleans – a pilot study. *American Annals of the Deaf,* **123**(8), 960–7.

Liljedahl, K. (1993). *Handikapp och omvärld – hundra års pedagogik för ett livslångt lärande, handicap and environment – a hundred years of pedagogical efforts aimed at lifelong learning.* Lund: Lund University.

Mar, H. and N. Sall (1995). Enhancing social opportunities and relationships of children who are deaf-blind. *Journal of Visual Impairment & Blindness,* **89**(3), 280–6.

Marschark, M. (2003). Cognitive functioning in deaf adults and children. In M. Marschark and P. E. Spencer, eds.

Oxford Handbook of Deaf Studies, Language and Education. Oxford: Oxford University Press, pp. 464–77.

McEwen, E. and H. Anton-Culver (1988). The medical communication of deaf patients. *Journal of Family Practice,* **26**(3), 289–91.

McInnes, J. and J. Treffry (1982). *Deaf-Blind Infants and Children. A Developmental Guide.* Milton Keynes: The Open University Press.

Meador, H. E. and P. Zazove (2005). Health care interactions with Deaf culture. *Journal of the American Board of Family Practice* **18**(3), 218–22.

Middleton, A. (2006). Genetic counselling and the d/Deaf community. In D. Stephens and L. Jones, eds. *The Effects of Genetic Hearing Impairment in the Family.* London: Wiley, pp. 257–84.

Middleton, A., S. Emery, et al. (2008). *Deafness and Genetics: What Do Deaf People Want?* Public Consultation, Millennium Centre, Cardiff Bay.

Middleton, A., J. Hewison, et al. (1998). Attitudes of deaf adults toward genetic testing for hereditary deafness. *American Journal of Human Genetics,* **63**, 1175–80.

Middleton, A., F. Robson, et al. (2007). Providing a transcultural genetic counseling service in the UK *Journal of Genetic Counseling,* **16**(5), 567–82.

Middleton, A., G. Turner, et al. (2009). Preferences for communication in clinic from deaf people: a cross-sectional study. *Journal of Evaluation in Clinical Practice* (in press).

Möller, C. (2007). Deafblindness. In A. Martini, D. Stephens and A. Read, eds. *Genes, Hearing and Deafness*. Oxford: Informa Healthcare, pp. 55–61.

Möller, K. (2008). *Impact on participation and service for persons with deafblindness*. Örebro: Örebro University.

Möller, K. and B. Danermark (2007). Social recognition, participation and the dynamics between the environment and personal factors of students with deafblindness. *American Annals of the Deaf,* **152**(1), 42–55.

Morton, C. and W. Nance (2006). Newborn hearing screening – a silent revolution. *New England Journal of Medicine,* **354**, 2151–64.

Morton, N. E. (1991). Genetic epidemiology of hearing impairment. *Annals of the New York Academy of Sciences,* **630**, 16–31.

Munoz-Baell, I. M. and M. T. Ruiz (2000). Empowering the deaf. Let the deaf be deaf. *Journal of Epidemiology and Community Health,* **54**, 40–4.

Myers, R. and A. Marcus (1993). Hearing. Mother, father deaf: issues of identity and mediation in culture and communication. *Deaf Studies III: Bridging Cultures in the 21st Century*. Washington DC: College for Continuing Education, Gallaudet University, pp. 171–84.

Nance, W., X. Liu, et al. (2000). Relation between choice of partner and high frequency of connexin 26 deafness. *Lancet,* **356**, 500–1.

Neary, W., D. Stephens, et al. (2006). Psychosocial aspects of Neurofibromatosis Type 2 reported by affected individuals. In D. Stephens and L. Jones, eds. *The Effects of Genetic Hearing Impairment in the Family.* Chichester: Wiley, pp. 207–36.

Newton, V. E. (1985). Aetiology of bilateral sensorineural hearing loss in young children. *Journal of Laryngology and Otology (Supplement)* **10**, 1–57.

NIH (1987, Jul 13–15). ''Neurofibromatosis Consens Statement Online. 6(12),1–19. Available at: http:// consensus.nih.gov/1987/1987Neurofibramatosis064html. htm. Retrieved 24 Feb 2009.

Nikolopoulos, T., Lioumi, et al. (2006). Evidence-based overview of ophthalmic disorders in deaf children: a literature update. *Otology & Neurotology,* **27**(2), S1–S24.

Padden, C. and T. Humphries (2005). *Inside Deaf Culture.* London: Harvard University Press.

Parving, A. (1983). Epidemiology of hearing loss and aetiological diagnosis of hearing impairment in childhood. *International Journal of Pediatric Otorhinolaryngology,* **5**, 151–65.

Parving, A. (1984). Aetiologic diagnosis in hearing-impaired children – clinical value and application of a modern programme. *International Journal of Pediatric Otorhinolaryngology,* **7**, 29–38.

Prosser, S. and A. Martini (2007). Understanding the phenotype: basic concepts in audiology. In A. Martini, D. Stephens and A. P. Read, eds. *Genes, Hearing and Deafness. From Molecular Biology to Clinical Practice.* London: Informa Healthcare, pp. 19–38.

Ralston, F. and J. Israel (1995). Language and communication. *An Introduction to Deafness: A Manual for Genetic Counselors.* Washington DC: Genetic Services Center, Gallaudet University.

Reardon, W. and M. Pembrey (1990). The genetics of deafness. *Archives of Disease in Childhood,* **65**, 1196–7.

Reeves, D. and B. Kokoruwe (2005). Communication and communication support in Primary care: a survey of deaf patients. *Audiological Medicine,* **3**, 95–107.

RNID (2004a). *The DDA – for Service Providers* (factsheet). London: Royal National Institute for Deaf People in-house publication.

RNID (2004b). *A Simple Cure.* London: Royal National Institute for Deaf People in-house publication.

RNID (2008). Statistics: deaf and hard of hearing adults in the UK. Retrieved 21 Feb 2008, from www.rnid.org.

Rogel, K. (2008). *Access to genetic services and education within the Deaf community.* MSc dissertation. New York: Sarah Lawrence College. p. 65.

Sadeghi, M. (2005). *Usher syndrome prevalence and phenotype-genotype correlations.* Göteborg: Göteborg University.

Schein, J. D. (1989). *At Home Amongst Strangers.* Washington DC: Gallaudet University Press.

Schiff-Myers, N. (1988). Hearing children of deaf parents. In D. Bishop and K. Mogford, eds. *Language Development in Exceptional Circumstances.* New York: Churchill pp. 47–61.

Schneider, J. (2006). *Becoming Deafblind: Negotiating a Place in a Hostile World.* Sydney: University of Sydney.

Schuchman, J. (2004). Deafness and eugenics in the Nazi era. In J. V. V. Cleve, ed. *Genetics, Disability and Deafness.* Washington DC: Gallaudet University Press.

Shaw, A. and M. Ahmed (2004). Translating genetic leaflets into languages other than English: lessons from an assessment of Urdu materials. *Journal of Genetic Counseling,* **13**(4), 321–42.

Smith, R. and Van Camp. (2008, 28/10/08). Deafness and hereditary hearing loss overview. Retrieved 19 Nov 2008, from http://www.ncbi.nlm.nih.gov.

Steinberg, A. G., S. Barnett, et al. (2006). Health care system accessibility: experiences and perceptions of deaf people. *Journal of General Internal Medicine,* **21**, 260–6.

Steinberg, A. G., V. J. Sullivan, et al. (1998). Cultural and linguistic barriers to mental health service access: the Deaf consumer's perspective. *American Journal of Psychiatry,* **155**(7), 982–4.

Stephens, D. (2005). The impact of hearing impairment in children. In D. Stephens and L. Jones, eds. *The Impact of Genetic Hearing Impairment.* London: Whurr, pp. 73–105.

Stephens, D. (2007). Psychosocial aspects of genetic hearing impairment. In A. Martini, D. Stephens and A. P. Read, eds. *Genes, Hearing and Deafness: From Molecular Biology to Clinical Practice.* London: Informa Healthcare, pp. 145–61.

Stephens, D. and B. Danermark (2005). The international classification of functioning, disability and health as a conceptual framework for the impact of genetic hearing impairment. In D. Stephens and L. Jones, eds. *The Impact of Genetic Hearing Impairment*. London: Whurr, pp. 54–67.

Stephens, D. and L. Jones, eds. (2005). *The Impact of Genetic Hearing Impairment*. London: Whurr.

Stephens, D. and L. Jones, eds. (2006). *The Effects of Genetic Hearing Impairment in the Family*. Chichester: Wiley.

Stephens, D., P. Lewis, et al. (2003). The influence of a perceived family history of hearing difficulties in an epidemiological study of hearing problems. *Audiological Medicine*, **1**, 228–31.

Toriello, H., W. Reardon, et al. (2004). *Hereditary Hearing Loss and Its Syndromes*. Oxford: Oxford University Press.

Ubido, J., J. Huntington, et al. (2002). Inequalities in access to healthcare faced by women who are deaf. *Health and Social Care in the Community*, **10**(4), 247–53.

Vernon, M. and J. Andrews (1990). Psychodynamics surrounding the diagnosis of deafness. In M. Vernon and J. Andrews, eds. *Psychology of Deafness – Understanding Deaf and Hard of Hearing People*. New York: Longman, pp. 119–36.

WFD (2009). World Federation of the Deaf homepage. Retrieved 26 Feb 2009, from http://www.wfdeaf.org/.

Wolf-Schein, E. (1989). A review of the size, characteristics, and needs of the deaf-blind population of North America. *ACEHI Journal*, **15**(3), 85–9.

Woll, B. and P. Ladd (2003). Deaf communities. In M. Marschark and P. E. Spencer, eds. *Oxford Handbook of Deaf Studies, Language and Education.* Oxford: Oxford University Press, pp. 151–63.

World Health Organization (2001). *International Classification of Functioning, Disability and Health (ICF).* Geneva: World Health Organization.

World Health Organization (2006). Deafness and hearing impairment. Retrieved 16th Mar 2009, from http://www.who.int/en/.

INDEX

Index

Index